Preventing coronary heart disease

The role of antioxidants, vegetables and fruit

Report of an expert meeting

Edited by

Lesley Rogers and Imogen Sharp

National Heart Forum
Tavistock House South
Tavistock Square
London WC1H 9LG

London: The Stationery Office

ISBN 0 11 322001 4

National Heart Forum
Tavistock House South
Tavistock Square
London WC1H 9LG

Registered Company Number: 2487644
Registered Charity Number: 803286
VAT Number: 564 6088 18

Other publications by the National Heart Forum:

At Least Five a Day: Strategies to Increase Vegetable and Fruit Consumption
Coronary Heart Disease Prevention in Undergraduate Medical Education
Coronary Heart Disease Prevention: A Catalogue of Key Resources
Coronary Heart Disease Prevention: Action in the UK 1984–1987
Coronary Heart Disease: Are Women Special?
Eat Your Words: Understanding Healthy Eating and Food Messages
Food For Children: Influencing Choice and Investing in Health
Physical Activity: An Agenda for Action
Preventing Coronary Heart Disease in Primary Care: The Way Forward
School Meals Assessment Pack

The Stationery Office

Published by The Stationery Office and available from:

The Publications Centre
(mail, telephone and fax orders only)
PO Box 276, London SW8 5DT
General enquiries 0171 873 0011
Telephone orders 0171 873 9090
Fax orders 0171 873 8200

The Stationery Office Bookshops
49 High Holborn, London WC1V 6HB
(counter service and fax orders only)
Fax 0171 831 1326
68-69 Bull Street, Birmingham B4 6AD
0121 236 9696 Fax 0121 236 9699
33 Wine Street, Bristol BS1 2BQ
0117 926 4306 Fax 0117 929 4515
9-21 Princess Street, Manchester M60 8AS
0161 834 7201 Fax 0161 833 0634
16 Arthur Street, Belfast BT1 4GD
01232 238451 Fax 01232 235401
The Stationery Office Oriel Bookshop
The Friary, Cardiff CF1 4AA
01222 395548 Fax 01222 384347
71 Lothian Road, Edinburgh EH3 9AZ
(counter service only)

Customers in Scotland may
mail, telephone or fax their orders to:
Scottish Publications Sales
South Gyle Crescent, Edinburgh EH12 9EB
0131 479 3141 Fax 0131 479 3142

Accredited Agents
(see Yellow Pages)

and through good booksellers

Acknowledgements

This report is based on a one-day expert meeting on *Antioxidant Nutrients, Fruit and Vegetables and the Prevention of Coronary Heart Disease,* held in March 1995. The National Heart Forum would like to thank all those who helped to organise and all those who participated in the meeting. Particular thanks are due to:

- The members of the Steering Group (see next page)

- All those who wrote or commented on papers in the original discussion document, the speakers who contributed papers, the session chairs, and all the other participants who contributed to the success of the expert meeting (see page v)

- Rosie Leyden (Wordworks) for editorial work on the report

- The Health Education Authority for financial assistance for the expert meeting and this report.

Steering Group

Dr Fleur Fisher (Chair)	British Medical Association
Mr Geoffrey Cannon	National Food Alliance and World Cancer Research Fund
Ms Anne Dillon Roberts	National Farmers Union
Ms Ann Foster	Scottish Consumer Council
Professor Desmond Julian	Chairman, National Heart Forum
Professor Michael Marmot	University College London
Dr Alan Maryon Davis	Faculty of Public Health Medicine
Professor Michael Oliver	National Heart and Lung Institute
Professor Brian Pentecost	British Heart Foundation
Ms Maggie Sanderson	British Dietetic Association and Honorary Secretary, National Heart Forum
Ms Imogen Sharp	Director, National Heart Forum
Ms Lynn Stockley	Health Education Authority
Ms Carmen Taboas	National Consumer Council
Ms Carol Williams	Nutrition Consultant
Dr Martin Wiseman	Department of Health
Dr John Yarnell	Health Promotion Agency for Northern Ireland

Meeting Coordinators

Dr Lesley Rogers	Assistant Director, National Heart Forum
Ms Jenni White	Project Officer, National Heart Forum

Contributors and participants

Dr Annie Anderson, Department of Human Nutrition, Glasgow Royal Infirmary

Dr Jane Armitage, Clinical Trial Service Unit, Radcliffe Infirmary, Oxford

Dr Margaret Ashwell, British Nutrition Foundation

Ms Mary Belizzi, Rowett Research Institute, Aberdeen

Dr Sheila Bingham,* Dunn Clinical Nutrition Centre, Cambridge

Dr Gladys Block,* Department of Social and Administrative Health Services, University of California, United States

Dr Eric Brunner, Department of Epidemiology and Public Health, University College London

Dr David Buss, Ministry of Agriculture, Fisheries and Food

Mr Geoffrey Cannon,* National Food Alliance/World Cancer Research Fund

Dr Rory Collins,* British Heart Foundation Research Fellow, Clinical Trial Service Unit, University of Oxford

Professor David de Bono, Academic Department of Cardiology, Glenfield Hospital, Leicester

Professor A T Diplock, Division of Biochemistry and Molecular Biology, United Medical and Dental School of Guy's and St Thomas's Hospitals, London

Dr David Gunnell, Department of Social Medicine, University of Bristol

Professor Barry Halliwell,* Pharmacology Group, King's College London

Professor W P T James,* The Rowett Research Institute, Aberdeen

Professor Desmond Julian, Chairman, National Heart Forum

Dr Dorian Kennedy, Ministry of Agriculture, Fisheries and Food

Professor Frans Kok, Department of Epidemiology and Public Health, Wageningen Agricultural University, Netherlands

Dr Daan Kromhout,* Division of Public Research, National Institute of Public Health & Environmental Protection, Netherlands

Professor Mike Lean, Department of Human Nutrition, Glasgow Royal Infirmary

Dr David Lindsay, Ministry of Agriculture, Fisheries and Food

Professor Michael Marmot, Department of Epidemiology and Public Health, University College London

Dr Paul McKeigue, Epidemiology Unit, London School of Hygiene and Tropical Medicine

Professor Klim McPherson, Health Promotion Sciences Unit, London School of Hygiene and Tropical Medicine, Honorary Treasurer, National Heart Forum

Professor Michael Oliver, Cardiac Medicine, National Heart and Lung Institute, London and Professor Emeritus, University of Edinburgh

Dr Ian O'Neill, Dunn Clinical Nutrition Centre, Cambridge

Dr Anne Payne, Cardiovascular Research Unit, University of Edinburgh

Dr Bruce Pearce, Ministry of Agriculture, Fisheries and Food

Professor Brian Pentecost, British Heart Foundation

Professor Catherine Rice-Evans, Free Radical Research Group, Division of Biochemistry, UMDS, University of London

Dr Rudolph Riemersma, Cardiovascular Research Unit, University of Edinburgh

Ms Sallie Robins, British Medical Association

Dr Lesley Rogers, Assistant Director, National Heart Forum

Ms Maggie Sanderson,* British Dietetic Association, Honorary Secretary, National Heart Forum

Ms Imogen Sharp,* Director, National Heart Forum

Ms Lynn Stockley, Health Education Authority

Dr Margaret Thorogood,* Health Promotion Sciences Unit, London School of Hygiene and Tropical Medicine

Professor David Thurnham,* School of Biomedical Science, University of Ulster

Professor Hugh Tunstall-Pedoe,* Cardiovascular Epidemiology Unit, Ninewells Hospital Medical School, Dundee

Ms Stephanie Whimpenny, Administrative Secretary, National Heart Forum

Ms Jenni White, Student Placement, National Heart Forum

Ms Carol Williams, Nutrition Consultant

Dr Martin Wiseman, Nutrition Unit, Department of Health

Dr John Yarnell, Department of Epidemiology and Public Health, Queen's University, Belfast

National Heart Forum

The National Heart Forum (formerly the National Forum for Coronary Heart Disease Prevention) is an alliance of over 35 national organisations concerned with the prevention of coronary heart disease. Members represent the health services, professional bodies, consumer groups and voluntary organisations.

The mission of the National Heart Forum is to work with and through its members to achieve a reduction in coronary heart disease mortality and morbidity rates throughout the UK. It has four main objectives:

- to keep under review the activities of member organisations and disseminate findings

- to identify areas of consensus, issues of controversy, and needs for action

- to facilitate the coordination of activities between interested organisations

- to make recommendations where appropriate.

Member organisations
ASH (Action on Smoking and Health)
Association for Public Health
Association of Facilitators in Primary Care
British Association for Cardiac Rehabilitation
British Cardiac Society
British Dietetic Association
British Heart Foundation
British Medical Association
British Nutrition Foundation
Chartered Institute of Environmental Health
Consumers' Association
CORDA
Coronary Prevention Group
Faculty of Public Health Medicine
Family Heart Association
Health Education Authority
Health Promotion Agency for Northern Ireland
Health Promotion Wales
Health Visitors' Association
National Association of Governors and Managers
National Association of Health Authorities and Trusts
Northern Ireland Chest, Heart and Stroke Association
Royal College of General Practitioners
Royal College of Nursing
Royal College of Paediatrics and Child Health

Royal College of Physicians of Edinburgh
Royal College of Physicians of London
Royal College of Surgeons of England
Royal Institute of Public Health and Hygiene
Royal Pharmaceutical Society of Great Britain
Society of Cardiothoracic Surgeons
Society of Health Education and Health Promotion Specialists
Society of Occupational Medicine
Sports Council
Trades Union Congress

Observers
Department of Health
Department of Health and Social Services, Northern Ireland
Medical Research Council
Ministry of Agriculture, Fisheries and Food
National Consumer Council
Scottish Consumer Council
Scottish Office, Home and Health Department
Welsh Office

In addition, a number of distinguished experts in the field have individual membership.

Contents

Foreword   **xi**

Part 1   **Summary and conclusions**   **1**

Part 2   **The scientific basis**   **9**

Chapter 1   Antioxidants and the development of coronary heart disease:
                the biological basis   11
                Professor A T Diplock and Dr Lesley A Rogers

Part 3   **The role of antioxidants and vegetables and fruit: the
                research evidence**   **17**

Chapter 2   Antioxidant nutrients and coronary heart disease: epidemiological,
                population and clinical trial evidence   19
                Professor Michael Oliver CBE

Chapter 3   Do vegetables and fruit protect against coronary heart
                disease? Studies among vegetarians   29
                Dr Margaret Thorogood

Chapter 4   Antioxidant nutrients and coronary heart disease:
                international evidence from the EURAMIC study   39
                Professor Frans Kok

Part 4   **Dietary recommendations on vegetables and fruit**   **47**

Chapter 5   Changing rationales, consistent advice: dietary
                recommendations on vegetables and fruit   49
                Carol Williams and Professor Michael Marmot

Chapter 6   At least five a day? Devising quantified dietary advice on
                vegetables and fruit   63
                Carol Williams and Professor Michael Marmot

Appendix   Rich sources of beta-carotene, vitamin C and vitamin E   73

Foreword

There is much interest among health professionals, policy makers and the public in the links between diet and disease. The focus has shifted recently to the possibility that increasing the intake of specific nutrients, such as antioxidants, could protect against major chronic diseases, including coronary heart disease and some cancers. Vegetables and fruit – the main dietary sources of antioxidant nutrients – have come under the spotlight.

This report explores the research evidence on the role of antioxidants and vegetables and fruit in reducing the risk of coronary heart disease. It derives from an expert meeting held by the National Heart Forum in 1995, which brought together over 40 experts from a range of disciplines – biological scientists, heart disease and cancer specialists, clinicians, epidemiologists, nutritionists, and policy makers responsible for developing and implementing dietary recommendations. The report also incorporates research evidence published since the expert meeting.

Credible policies should be based on scientific consensus, so this report focuses on the science on which policy options can be built. It considers the biological mechanisms by which antioxidants may lower the risk of coronary heart disease; evidence from epidemiological and clinical studies on the role of antioxidant nutrients, vitamin supplements and vegetables and fruit in lowering the risk of coronary heart disease; consumption patterns of antioxidant nutrients and fruit and vegetables in the UK; and national and international dietary recommendations for preventing coronary heart disease as well as cancer.

The report outlines the evidence, highlights areas of uncertainty and sets out the conclusions of the expert meeting:

- Evidence for a protective effect of specific antioxidants, particularly vitamins E and C and beta-carotene, is incomplete; further research is needed before recommendations for specific antioxidants can be made.

- There is good evidence that a diet rich in a range of vegetables and fruit is beneficial and lowers the risk of coronary heart disease.

- National and international recommendations to increase fruit and vegetable intakes to at least five portions a day form a sound basis for policy.

There is strong scientific evidence to support an increase in intakes of vegetables and fruit in the UK. But further research is needed to clarify which particular components of fruit and vegetables are responsible for their protective effects. Until more is known about the precise effects of antioxidants and of other bioactive micronutrients in vegetables and fruit, it is appropriate to raise the intakes of antioxidant nutrients by increasing the consumption of vegetables and fruit rather than through vitamin supplements. A focus on antioxidant vitamin supplements is not only inappropriate in light of the evidence, but also likely to shift attention away from the need for overall improvements in the UK's diet.

We hope that this report, generously funded by the Health Education Authority, will contribute to a better understanding of the scientific basis on the role of antioxidants and vegetables and fruit in preventing coronary heart disease, and pave the way for improvements in public health.

A second National Heart Forum report, *At Least Five a Day: Strategies to Increase Vegetable and Fruit Consumption,* sets out policy recommendations developed from this scientific base. Targeted strategies to reach the goal of 'at least five a day' in the UK now need to be implemented.

Professor Desmond Julian CBE MD FRCP
Chairman, National Heart Forum

Part I

Summary and conclusions

Summary and conclusions

MAIN CONCLUSIONS

- Evidence for a protective effect of specific antioxidants, particularly vitamins E and C and beta-carotene, is incomplete; further research is needed before recommendations for specific antioxidants can be made.

- There is good evidence that a diet rich in a range of vegetables and fruit is beneficial and lowers the risk of coronary heart disease.

- National and international recommendations to increase fruit and vegetable intakes to at least five portions a day form a sound basis for policy.

Antioxidant nutrients, free radicals and the development of coronary heart disease

Is the scientific evidence convincing? Are the mechanisms biologically plausible?

Free radicals – highly reactive oxygen molecules – are involved in many processes essential to the efficient functioning of the body, including the secretion of hormones, muscle contraction and in the body's defence system against bacteria and tumour cells. However, there is evidence that they play a role in the development of coronary heart disease, including angina and myocardial infarction (heart attack).

The most convincing and biologically plausible link between free radicals, antioxidant nutrients and coronary heart disease centres on evidence that free radicals can damage or oxidise low density lipoprotein (LDL) cholesterol. The effect on other processes, such as cell proliferation and cell death, is less clear. (See Chapter 1.)

Antioxidant nutrients, the best known of which are vitamins C and E and beta-carotene*, appear to be able to help control damage by free radicals, at least in experimental model systems in the laboratory. This is particularly so for vitamin E. However, the exact mechanism by which antioxidants may protect against the development of coronary heart disease remains uncertain.

More evidence is needed on the stages in the development of coronary heart disease and cancer at which free radicals and antioxidant nutrients act. Research is also needed to tease out the significance of, as well as any links between, damage caused by free radicals and other risk factors for disease including smoking, other nutritional factors, physical activity, and social and genetic variations in humans.

- **The link between damage caused by free radicals and the protective effect of antioxidant nutrients in the development of coronary heart disease and cancers in experimental animal models is biologically robust and forms a useful working model. However, the exact mechanism by which antioxidants may protect against the development of coronary heart disease remains uncertain.**

Evidence from epidemiological studies and clinical trials

Is the evidence convincing? What are the implications for the population?

Antioxidant nutrients
A number of studies have shown that low intakes of antioxidant nutrients, particularly vitamins E and C, are related to higher rates of coronary heart disease. These studies include cross-sectional studies, case control studies and intervention trials. (See Chapter 2).

Although there are some exceptions, cross-sectional studies comparing different populations within one country or between different countries in Europe have generally found that those populations with a high incidence of coronary heart disease have lower plasma levels of vitamin E and to a lesser extent vitamin C. Similar patterns have been found for other substances with antioxidant properties, such as the flavonoids present in vegetables, fruits, tea and wine.

The effect of antioxidant vitamin supplements has been examined in a number of studies. Two large observational studies in the United States, one among nurses and one among male health professionals, examined the effects of intakes of vitamins E and C and beta-carotene, from diet and supplements, on rates of coronary heart disease. Both found that those who took vitamin E supplements had a lower incidence of coronary heart disease. Cautious interpretation is needed however, because those people taking vitamin supplements were also less likely to smoke, more likely to be physically active and, in the case of nurses, to be taking hormone replacement therapy, compared with those in the study who did not take supplements. Thus, it is

---

*   For details of rich dietary sources of these vitamins, see the Appendix.

possible that the lower rates of coronary heart disease were due to other lifestyle factors. In the male health professionals study, there was no association between the incidence of coronary heart disease and beta-carotene or vitamin C intakes. While these results are interesting, it is hard to extrapolate to the general population because the study groups differ in many ways. (See Chapter 2.)

Several case control studies have examined levels of antioxidant nutrients in blood or adipose tissue in people who have suffered a heart attack or angina, compared with those in a healthy control group. In these studies, it was rare for participants to take vitamin supplements, so antioxidant levels in tissues were considered to result from diet. One major study across Europe, the EURAMIC study, found little or no evidence for a protective effect from vitamin E. However, very low levels of beta-carotene, especially in current and ex-smokers, were associated with an increased risk of coronary heart disease. (See Chapter 4.)

Randomised controlled trials are generally viewed as the 'gold standard' when assessing the effects of antioxidants. Several controlled trials of vitamin supplements have been published. One such study, in Finland, examined the effect of beta-carotene supplements with and without vitamin E supplements on death rates from coronary heart disease and lung cancer in middle aged male smokers. There was no difference in death rates from coronary heart disease between those taking vitamin E and the controls. However, men taking beta-carotene had *higher* rates of death from coronary heart disease and lung cancer than the controls. These findings received support more recently in a study in the United States. The Beta-Carotene and Retinol Efficacy Trial (CARET), a study of beta-carotene combined with vitamin A (retinol) supplements in men and women at risk of lung cancer through smoking or extensive occupational exposure to asbestos, found that, after four years of supplementation, there was an increased risk of both cardiovascular disease and lung cancer. As a result, the study was terminated 21 months early.

The possibility that antioxidant nutrients may lower risk in patients with confirmed coronary heart disease is also being investigated. Results from the Cambridge Heart Antioxidant Study (CHAOS) suggested that patients who took vitamin E supplements for less than two years had lower rates of non-fatal myocardial infarction, but cardiovascular deaths were marginally, but not significantly, higher in patients taking vitamin E than in the control group.

Both the epidemiological evidence and that of observational studies, for example the Finnish survey and the Iowa Women's Health Study, suggest an inverse relationship between dietary vitamin E intake and coronary heart disease mortality: higher levels of intake are associated with lower mortality. (See Chapter 2.)

- **The picture which emerges from the studies of antioxidants is mixed. There is some evidence that populations with lower rates of coronary heart disease have higher plasma levels of vitamin E and, to a lesser extent, vitamin C. In observational studies, there is some evidence of benefit from higher intakes of vitamin E from food and supplements. However, cautious interpretation is needed because those taking supplements also tend to be healthier in other ways. Importantly, none of the long-term** clinical trials of antioxidant supplements have shown a reduction in coronary heart disease mortality. Furthermore, there is some evidence of harm, with an increased risk of cardiovascular disease and lung cancer among those taking beta-carotene and vitamin A supplements, and particularly in populations at high risk, such as smokers.

- **It is too early to make recommendations on vitamin supplements as a means of protecting populations at high or low risk of coronary heart disease. There is not clear enough evidence of benefit, and there is evidence of the possible harmful effect of certain vitamin supplements. Large scale and long-term randomised controlled trials are needed.**

What are the implications for the population?
It is still very uncertain how these research findings relate to the general population.

Beta-carotene is one of several hundred carotenoids and its absorption in the gut depends on transport systems about which little is known. It is possible that large doses of beta-carotene compete with other carotenoids with different antioxidant effects, for transport into the body, and block their absorption. As a result, selected beta-carotene supplements may increase the chance of certain chronic diseases developing.

The relationship between levels of specific antioxidants in blood or adipose tissue and intakes of vegetables and fruit also remains uncertain. Fruit and vegetables contain many different types of antioxidants and other nutrients. It is possible that those antioxidants which have been studied are simply markers for other essential nutrients in fruit and vegetables yet to be identified. These components may act together and have a multiplicative or synergistic effect, which supplements cannot necessarily replicate.

Fruit and vegetables
Several studies have investigated whether a diet rich in fruit and vegetables protects against coronary heart disease. These studies generally lend positive support to the hypothesis, although as yet there is little direct evidence. While there are cross-sectional data, there is a lack of intervention and trial data on the effects of a diet rich in fruit and vegetables on rates of coronary heart disease. The evidence in relation to cancer is stronger and more readily available. (See Chapter 5.)

It has been difficult to obtain accurate and comprehensive data on fruit and vegetable intakes in either observational or case control studies. A number of studies have focused on populations with diets rich in vegetables and fruit, such as vegetarians and Seventh Day Adventists. However, these groups often differ from the general population in other important ways. For example, vegetarians tend to smoke less, are less likely to be overweight and tend to come from social classes I and II - all of which confer a health advantage. In addition, diets rich in vegetables and fruit also tend to be lower in saturated fat.

Furthermore, just as antioxidant levels measured in epidemiological and clinical studies may be markers for other factors in plant-based foods, so fruit and vegetable intakes may also be markers not only for antioxidant nutrients but also for other, yet to be identified, bioactive micronutrients with a protective effect. (See Chapter 5.)

- The strong message emerging from the studies of diets rich in fruit and vegetables is that they are associated with lower overall death rates and death rates from coronary heart disease. Evidence that such diets also protect against some cancers strengthens the support for recommendations to increase vegetable and fruit consumption. There is no evidence that such diets cause harm.

Dietary recommendations and current intakes

Antioxidant nutrients

The scientific evidence currently available leaves uncertainty about the role specific antioxidant nutrients may play in the development of coronary heart disease.

Vegetables, fruits and fruit juice are the main dietary sources of vitamin C and beta-carotene, and these provide about 80% of vitamin C and 70% of beta-carotene. Rich sources of vitamin E also include vegetable oils and nuts as well as fruit and vegetables. (See Appendix.)

Intakes of antioxidant nutrients in the UK vary by social class, age and geographic region. The lowest dietary intakes of vitamin C, beta-carotene and vitamin E tend to be found in Scotland and among socioeconomic groups IV and V; the highest in London and the South East and in socioeconomic groups I and II. Cigarette smokers also eat fewer vegetables and fruit and have a low intake of the two main antioxidant vitamins E and C.

The average population intake of vitamin C and E meets the current recommended UK Reference Nutrient Intake (RNI); there is no RNI for beta-carotene. However, RNIs are currently set at levels to protect against clinical deficiencies, rather than to protect against chronic diseases such as coronary heart disease. (See Chapter 6.)

- There is insufficient evidence to recommend which type or how much of each antioxidant nutrient might lower the risk of coronary heart disease.

- Considering all the evidence available, it would be premature to make recommendations for population-wide intakes of selected antioxidants in order to lower the risk of coronary heart disease.

Fruit and vegetables

On the basis of the research evidence, a number of international and national agencies, including the World Health Organization (WHO), the Committee on Medical Aspects of Food Policy (COMA) Cardiovascular Review Group, and the Working Party which produced *The Scottish Diet* report, have all concluded that fruit and vegetable intakes should be increased (see Chapter 5). The WHO recommends an average population intake of at least 400g of fruit and vegetables every day. *The Scottish Diet* report recommends a doubling of fruit and vegetable consumption to at least 400g a day, and COMA recommended that consumption of vegetables, fruit, potatoes and bread increase by at least 50%. The recommendations are consistent and support advice on intakes of at least five portions of fruit and vegetables (excluding potatoes) each day.

Average consumption of vegetables and fruit in the UK, in 1994, was about 250g a day – or three portions. However, there are large social class and regional variations, and over a third of the population eat less than 250g each day. For example, average daily intakes in Scotland are 180g. Even those social groups with the highest intakes, socioeconomic groups I and II, eat only 300g of fruit and vegetables a day.

There has been only a gradual increase in the consumption of fruit and vegetables in the UK in the last 30 years. This increase has been mainly due to increases in frozen vegetables, salad vegetables, fruit juices and citrus fruit.

- **The national and international recommendations to increase average vegetable and fruit consumption levels to at least 400g each day – equivalent to five portions a day – form a sound basis for policy. Increasing vegetable and fruit consumption levels towards this goal would help reduce the risk of coronary heart disease, as well as cancer.**

Research needs

Although there are several research programmes and studies underway, more research is needed in the following areas:

- the link between free radicals and the biological events occurring during the development of coronary heart disease

- the relationship between levels of antioxidant nutrients in the blood and levels in adipose tissue, and how these relate to intake

- case control studies on the antioxidant nutrient status of angina patients

- the effect of antioxidant nutrients with and without pharmacological interventions, such as cholesterol-lowering drugs, in people with evidence of coronary heart disease

- the range and variety of antioxidant nutrients present in different foods, including whether the protective effect of the 'Mediterranean diet' is due to the variety and/or amount of antioxidant nutrients consumed

- the effect of different methods of storage, processing and cooking on the nutrient content of fruit and vegetables

- effective interventions to increase fruit and vegetable intakes – including interventions which address individual behaviour change and issues of availability and access. Population interventions need to take account of social and regional variations.

The challenge ahead

Building on this scientific consensus, strategies now need to be developed to increase vegetable and fruit intakes in the UK to meet the goal of at least 400g or at least five portions a day. A second National Heart Forum expert meeting addressed these issues, and the report *At Least Five a Day: Strategies to Increase Vegetable and Fruit Consumption*, sets out its recommendations. The challenge ahead is to implement the strategies for change.

Part 2

The scientific basis

Antioxidants and the development of coronary heart disease: the biological basis

Professor A T Diplock

Division of Biochemistry and Molecular Biology, United Medical and Dental School of Guy's and St Thomas's Hospitals, London

Dr Lesley A Rogers

National Heart Forum

Introduction

The latest Committee on Medical Aspects of Food Policy report on *Nutritional Aspects of Cardiovascular Disease* highlights the link between dietary factors and cardiovascular disease, including coronary heart disease.[1] This link is supported by a substantial, diverse and generally consistent body of evidence. Furthermore, there is now a convincing picture of the mechanisms by which some dietary factors may cause or exacerbate the disease process and other factors in the diet appear to be protective.

There is some evidence that antioxidant nutrients, in particular, may lower the risk of major diseases, including coronary heart disease and certain cancers. This section focuses on the mechanism on which these nutrients may lower the risk of coronary heart disease, by neutralising or attenuating the effect of highly reactive molecules called 'free radicals', which seem to play a role in the development of coronary heart disease.

The main antioxidant nutrients which may have a protective effect are the vitamins E and C, the carotenoids (particularly beta-carotene) and the trace mineral selenium.* These are found in a very wide range of foods of plant origin. Good sources include fruits (especially citrus fruit) and vegetables, whole grain cereals and some vegetable oils. Other carotenoids such as lutein and lycopenes found in large amounts in tomatoes, and the flavonoids present in red wine, tea and onions, have also been implicated in lowering the risk of disease.**

---

*   The definition of vitamins E and C, the carotenoids and selenium as antioxidant nutrients is for convenience only; it may not be strictly valid, because it assumes that the function in disease prevention of these nutrients is that of an antioxidant. This may be true in some instances, but these nutrients may lower the risk of disease through other mechanisms also.

** It should be noted that beta-carotene is one of many carotenoids present in food. Lutein, a hydroxycarotenoid, is commonly found in equal, if not greater amounts in blood than beta-carotene. The flavonoids, which are widespread in fruits and vegetables, may also play an important role, but few studies have addressed their properties because of analytical deficiencies.

A diet rich in vegetables and fruits, and therefore rich in dietary antioxidants, may protect against the development of coronary heart disease in a number of ways. The main mechanism, discussed in this chapter, is the role antioxidant nutrients play in counteracting the effect of free radicals.

Coronary heart disease

The term coronary heart disease represents a number of different clinical conditions such as angina, myocardial infarction (heart attack) or sudden death. There is general consensus that the clinical manifestations of coronary heart disease are caused by a combination of atherosclerosis and thrombosis (see box below.)

The damage to the walls of the arteries, the build-up of fatty deposits in the blood vessels and the formation of fatty streaks and plaques, may all take years to develop. The causes and mechanisms by which these changes occur may also be varied and complex. However, it is becoming generally accepted that free radicals play a role in the underlying biochemical events involved in atherosclerosis,[2] and that antioxidant nutrients may help to control these events.

Summary of main events in the development of coronary heart disease

Atherosclerosis is a condition in which the lining of the arteries becomes thickened in places. This is caused by the deposition of raised plaques formed where modified lipid and smooth muscle cells, which are derived from within the arterial wall, have gathered. The size and severity of atherosclerotic lesions vary, from areas of lipid accumulation, called 'fatty streaks', to mature plaques.

Types of white blood cells, called macrophages, develop within the arterial walls into 'foam cells' when they take up chemically damaged or modified low density lipoprotein (LDL). These 'foam cells' develop into fatty streaks, some of which may progress to become atherosclerotic plaques.

Atherosclerotic plaques grow as more lipid is deposited and the smooth muscle cells in the plaque are stimulated to proliferate. The plaques then narrow the artery and restrict blood flow. This can result in angina or sudden death. If the delicate vessel wall lining, or endothelium, is damaged, other blood cells such as platelets are attracted to and gather at the site of the damage. Here they release a cocktail of chemicals which stimulate cell growth, inhibit the relaxation of the vessel walls, and attract more cells to the damaged vessel forming a clot or thrombus.

The formation of a large thrombus from platelet aggregation at the site of an atherosclerotic plaque can block the artery and lead to acute myocardial infarction (heart attack) or stroke, depending on the site of the blocked vessel. In the majority of cases, this blockage is started by a tear or split through the plaque, releasing the potent mixture of chemicals and cells.

What are free radicals and what role do they play in coronary heart disease?

It is customary to think of oxygen as a benign, life-giving substance upon which animals depend. Paradoxically, although oxygen is vital to life – it is essential in the release of energy from food – it can also be lethal. This is because oxygen molecules readily convert into several different chemical forms, known as 'free radicals', that are chemically much more reactive than the oxygen molecules present in the air. When the reactivity of these molecules is harnessed and controlled, they have important uses in the body. Controlled reactions involving free radicals are a normal part of many biological processes. However, uncontrolled free radical reactions can damage tissues and lead to disease.

Free radicals are involved in many processes which are essential to the efficient functioning of the body. These reactions include the contraction of muscles and the secretion of hormones. In addition, free radicals form a key part of the body's defence system against bacteria and tumour cells. An important mechanism by which oxygen and other free radicals are kept in check involves antioxidant nutrients.

What are free radicals?

A 'free radical' is an atom or molecule with one or more unpaired electron in their structure. Some free radicals are unstable and highly reactive.

Oxygen and hydrogen atoms consist of a positively charged nucleus which is surrounded by negatively charged electrons. The electrons are in orbit around the nucleus rather like satellites around a planet. Atoms are most stable, and least reactive, when the electrons they contain are paired and each member of the pair orbits the nucleus in opposite directions. If the electrons become unpaired, forming a free radical, the atom or molecule is more reactive than when the electrons are paired.

If the free radical is highly reactive, such as some of the free radicals formed in chemical reactions involving water or oxygen molecules, they may attack other non-radical molecules. The by-products of these reactions may themselves be unstable, reactive free radicals.

Polyunsaturated lipids may be oxidised by a staged process that involves free radicals. The first step which results in the formation of a new free radical is called *initiation*. The formation of further free radicals from other lipid molecules, which in turn react with stable molecules in a self-perpetuating chain reaction, is called the *propagation* phase. This chain reaction can potentially do much damage until the chain is *terminated* when all unpaired electrons become paired or stable.

When oxygen is reduced to water the superoxide anion radical, hydrogen peroxide and the hydroxyl radical may be formed. The hydroxyl radical, and lipid-derived peroxyl and alkoxyl radicals are the most biologically important and potent free radicals implicated in disease processes.

Targets for attack by free radicals

There are three principal targets for attack by free radicals in living cells: DNA, proteins and polyunsaturated fatty acids. The main link between free radical mediated cell damage and coronary heart disease is through oxidative damage to the polyunsaturated fatty acids in LDL cholesterol.

Polyunsaturated fatty acids

Unsaturated fatty acids are found in cell membranes as well as in the circulating LDL cholesterol molecules. The chemical structure of these molecules makes them attractive targets for free radical attack. The lipid peroxides formed when free radicals attack polyunsaturated fatty acids may be further degraded giving rise to products which are biologically active.

Proteins

The damage to polyunsaturated fatty acids by free radicals is the key link between free radicals, coronary heart disease and antioxidant nutrients. The products of free radical damage to lipids, the lipid hydroperoxides, can be degraded to small molecules that can also alter the structure and function of proteins. However, direct damage by free radicals to certain amino acids within proteins is also known to occur. If the protein is an enzyme it may no longer be able to catalyse reactions efficiently. If the protein plays a key role in the structure of the cell, damage may have widespread detrimental consequences leading to cell death.

The oxidation of LDL

There is substantial evidence from epidemiological, clinical and laboratory studies that the higher the level of cholesterol in the blood, the higher the risk of coronary heart disease mortality. Populations with higher mean plasma cholesterol levels generally have higher coronary heart disease death rates. Plasma cholesterol is made up of a number of different subfractions. The majority of cholesterol is carried in LDL cholesterol and it is high levels of this type of cholesterol, in the blood in particular, which has a positive relationship with risk of coronary heart disease. Low levels of LDL cholesterol correspond with reduced risk of coronary heart disease. The LDL cholesterol molecule is complex comprising: a cholesterol ester core surrounded by phospholipids (including polyunsaturated fatty acids), protein (called apoB$_{100}$) and cholesterol molecules. In addition the fat soluble vitamin E, and beta-carotene, are also contained within the LDL cholesterol complex. It is the phospholipid part of the LDL cholesterol which is most prone to damage by free radicals. It is thought that the balance of antioxidant nutrients in the LDL cholesterol complex may be critical for its protection from free radical attack.[3]

There are at least two consequences of the oxidation (ie chemical alteration) of polyunsaturated fatty acids in LDL cholesterol by free radicals:

1   Lipid free radicals are formed as a by-product of the reaction, and degradation products of these modify the apoprotein B so that it is recognised by macrophages within the arterial wall.

2   The oxidatively damaged LDL cholesterol is preferentially taken up by the macrophages, which then become trapped within the arterial wall, leading to fatty streak formation.

Most cells in the body have receptors which can bind LDL cholesterol, taking it out of the circulation. This is the principal mechanism of delivery of cholesterol from the liver, where it is synthesised, to peripheral tissues. However, these receptors cannot recognise and bind LDL cholesterol which has been oxidised, or modified in other ways, by free radicals. By contrast, the receptors on macrophages preferentially bind modified LDL cholesterol. When the macrophages become overladen with modified LDL cholesterol they form the 'foam cells' found in atherosclerotic lesions.

Prevention of free radical attack by antioxidants

A series of complex control mechanisms are thought to hold free radicals in check. Many of these mechanisms depend on an adequate supply of antioxidant nutrients in the diet. Antioxidant nutrients may act at two stages:

1   The prevention of *initiation*. Antioxidant minerals, that are part of enzyme structures, inactivate free radicals before they have a chance to initiate an oxidation chain reaction.

2   The prevention of *propagation*. Chain-breaking antioxidants interfere with an oxidation chain once it has started by trapping free radicals and terminating the reaction.

There are three main lines of defence, operating at the stages outlined above, against damage caused by free radicals.

- The first involves enzymes such as superoxide dismutases and glutathione peroxidases, which break down hydrogen peroxide. These enzymes prevent the proliferation of oxygen free radicals, and need trace minerals, such as selenium, copper and zinc, to function efficiently.

- The second comprises the lipid antioxidants, mainly vitamin E, which may function in concert with vitamin C, and the carotenoids. These block the formation of lipid hydroperoxides within lipoprotein molecules such as the LDL cholesterol complex.

- The third involves the removal of lipid hydroperoxides by selenium-containing glutathione peroxidases.

Vitamins E, C and beta-carotene

The antioxidant nutrient which is thought to play the most important role in controlling the process of LDL cholesterol oxidation is vitamin E. Vitamin E and beta-carotene are fat soluble nutrients. A large part of the plasma vitamin E is found in the LDL in the blood. Other antioxidants are present in the blood in much smaller concentrations. Since vitamin E is able to form a close association with the polyunsaturated fatty acid molecules it is therefore in a prime position to break free radical initiated chain reactions. Vitamin C (ascorbic acid) is water soluble and it is possible that it converts vitamin E, which has reacted with lipid peroxyl radicals, back to an active form able to block the further action of lipid radicals. This synergistic effect between vitamins E and C needs further study since some experimental animal studies have shown that vitamin E can be regenerated in the absence of vitamin C.

Until recently it was thought that the sole function of the carotenoids, such as beta-carotene, was to act as a precursor for vitamin A. Nevertheless quite substantial amounts of carotenoids can be absorbed from the diet, without being changed to vitamin A. Carotenoids have been shown to be capable of acting as antioxidants in experimental animal studies, but their role in preventing coronary heart disease development is unclear. Studies by Gey et al[4] have suggested that beta-carotene may be able to protect against atherosclerosis.

Selenium

Trace amounts of minerals such as selenium are needed for the optimal functioning of metal ion-dependent enzymes. These enzymes control the formation and proliferation of oxygen-derived free radicals and they also catalyse the removal of lipid hydroperoxides. However, studies of blood selenium levels and coronary heart disease death rates have been equivocal.

Conclusion

Laboratory and human epidemiological studies tend to support the general hypothesis that antioxidant nutrients may help lower the risk of coronary heart disease. The strongest evidence for this is to be found in relation to vitamins E and C, and beta-carotene, and the trace mineral selenium. Of these antioxidant nutrients, it is the enhancement of the vitamin E content of lipoproteins which seems to slow down the process of LDL cholesterol oxidation by free radicals, and consequently may possibly lower the risk of developing coronary heart disease. Further laboratory and intervention studies may clarify the type, amount and mechanism by which antioxidant nutrients lower the risk of coronary heart disease.

References

1   Department of Health. 1994. *Nutritional Aspects of Cardiovascular Disease. Report of the Cardiovascular Review Group, Committee on Medical Aspects of Food Policy. Report on Health and Social Subjects 46.* London: HMSO.
2   Steinberg D. 1992. Antioxidants in the prevention of human atherosclerosis. Summary of the proceedings of a National Heart, Lung and Blood Institute Workshop: September 5-6, 1991, Bethesda, Maryland. *Circulation*: 85 (6): 2337-2344.
3   Witzum DL. 1994. The oxidation hypothesis of atherosclerosis. *Lancet*; 344: 793-795.
4   Gey KF, Brubacher GM, Stahelin HB. 1987. Plasma levels of antioxidant vitamins in relation to ischemic heart disease and cancer. *American Journal of Clinical Nutrition*; 45: 1368-1377.

This paper derives from a monograph: Diplock AT. 1994. Antioxidants and disease prevention. In: *Molecular Aspects of Disease*: 15 (4). London: Pergamon Press.

Part 3

The role of antioxidants and vegetables and fruit: the research evidence

Antioxidant nutrients and coronary heart disease: epidemiological, population and clinical trial evidence

Professor Michael Oliver CBE

Cardiac Medicine, National Heart and Lung Institute, London

Introduction

In recent years it has been recognised that free radical formation may be causally related to both coronary heart disease and cancer.

Free radicals are a chemical species with one or more unpaired electrons. The most harmful free radicals are unpaired oxygen (stable molecules contain paired electrons), hydroperoxides and superoxide anions. Free radicals develop widely in human cells but are precisely controlled by several antioxidant protective mechanisms[1] including both enzymes and stabilising substances in the diet, such as vitamin E, vitamin C, beta carotene and vitamin A. An unbalanced excess of free radicals due to a lack of antioxidants could increase the risk of coronary heart disease in several ways, such as increasing the susceptibility of low density lipoproteins to undergo oxidation, increasing platelet adhesiveness, adversely influencing arterial endothelial function and impeding the repair of ischaemic myocardial damage.[2–5] (See Chapter 1 for further details.)

Evidence that low intakes of antioxidants may be relevant to the development of coronary heart disease comes from four sources – epidemiological data, case control studies, observational surveys in selected populations, and controlled trials.

Epidemiology

Epidemiological data suggest that the incidence of coronary heart disease, particularly in Europe, is inversely related to the plasma levels of vitamin E (alpha-tocopherol) and, to a lesser extent, to vitamin C. Countries with a very high incidence of coronary heart disease, such as Scotland, Northern Ireland

and Finland, have significantly lower plasma levels of vitamin E (alpha-tocopherol), and the Mediterranean countries have a low incidence of coronary heart disease with a relatively high consumption of antioxidant vitamins.[6]

A European cross-sectional survey of middle-aged men examined the relationship between plasma concentrations of vitamin E (alpha-tocopherol) and death rates from coronary heart disease.[7] The survey, although not random in sampling and not necessarily representative of the populations under study, was based on the known excess of deaths from coronary heart disease in northern countries. This study found a significant inverse correlation between plasma concentrations of vitamin E (alpha-tocopherol, lipid standardised) and death rates from coronary heart disease: death rates were higher in those populations with low plasma concentrations of vitamin E (alpha-tocopherol). A weaker inverse association with coronary heart disease deaths was found for for vitamin C. When vitamin E (alpha-tocopherol) and vitamin C were considered together, the inverse correlation was more marked.

In the UK, there are marked differences in vitamin E intake. Those in the least privileged sections of the community have particularly low intakes of vitamin E and vitamin C, due to their poor nutrition in terms of vegetables and fruit. Thus, the OPCS *Dietary and Nutritional Survey of British Adults*[8] found marked differences in the ratio of plasma vitamin E (alpha-tocopherol) concentration to serum cholesterol level, with lowest ratios in the north of England, social classes IV and V, and the unemployed (see Table 1). These differences were most marked in urban communities.

Table 1 *Average vitamin E (alpha-tocopherol)/cholesterol ratios in the UK*

Region	London/ South East	Central/West	North	Scotland	
	4.72 ± 0.06	4.70 ± 0.06	4.52 ± 0.08	4.56 ± 0.13	P<0.05
Social class	I & II	III	IV & V		
	4.83 ± 0.07	4.35 ± 0.06	4.41 ± 0.08		P<0.01
Work status	In work	Unemployed			
	4.73 ± 0.04	4.08 ± 0.10			P<0.01
Smoking habits	Non-smokers	1–20 cigarettes/day	>20 cigarettes/day		
	4.82 ± 0.05	4.41 ± 0.09	4.22 ± 0.08		P<0.01

See reference 8.

A relatively low intake of antioxidant vitamins, especially in smokers, probably contributes to the higher incidence of coronary heart disease in the north of England and Scotland. Cigarette smokers eat fewer vegetables and fruit and have a low intake of the two main antioxidant vitamins E and C.[9] The OPCS Survey showed that those who smoked more than 20 cigarettes daily had a lower ratio than that of non-smokers. Part of the explanation of the positive relationship between smoking and coronary heart disease may therefore be dietary.

Preventing coronary heart disease. The role of antioxidants, vegetables and fruit

The potent antioxidant activity of phenolic substances in red wine has been proposed as a protective mechanism to slow the development of atherosclerosis by reducing the oxidation of LDL cholesterol.[10] Indeed, this has been put forward as an explanation of the French 'paradox' of low coronary heart disease rates in a country with a high consumption of animal fat and excess cigarette smoking. There is no doubt concerning the increase in serum antioxidant activity after drinking red wine.[10]

The Scottish Heart Health Study[11] examined excess coronary risk and frequency of consumption of different foods, including fruit and vegetables, in 10,359 men and women aged 40-59. Among men with the highest coronary mortality (SMR 136), 17% ate no green vegetables and 30% ate no fruit. These figures contrast with those who had the lowest coronary mortality (SMR 61), of whom 6% ate no green vegetables and 13% ate no fruit.

Case control study: angina and myocardial infarction

A case control study[12] was carried out among people with angina of recent onset and controls, derived from a population of 6,000 men with a high incidence of coronary heart disease in Scotland. This study found that the risk of developing angina was strongly related to low plasma concentrations of vitamin E (alpha-tocopherol)/cholesterol and, to a lesser extent, vitamin C and beta-carotene (see Table 2). No correlation was found for vitamin A. A similar relationship has been demonstrated for patients with a first myocardial infarction and no previous angina. The relationship between low vitamin E (alpha-tocopherol) and these clinical manifestations of coronary heart disease was independent of cigarette smoking, although the levels of all the antioxidant vitamins were lower in smokers. The effect of smoking on vitamin C levels was particularly marked.

Table 2 *Relative risk of angina pectoris in a healthy male population*

	Quintiles of plasma concentrations in control population (n=382)				
	1 (low)	2	3	4	5 (high)
Vitamin E (alpha-tocopherol)/cholesterol	2.2*	1.8	1.1	1.1	1.0
Vitamin C	1.6	1.3	1.6	0.9	1.0
Beta-carotene	1.4	1.0	1.0	1.0	1.0

105 cases of new angina and 382 controls
All risk ratios were adjusted by logistic regression for age, smoking, blood pressure, cholesterol, LDL cholesterol, HDL cholesterol, triglycerides, relative weight and season.
* P <0.02
Source: See reference 12.

Observational studies

Several large observational studies have investigated the relationship between antioxidant nutrients in the diet, or vitamin supplements, and the incidence of coronary heart disease.

Dietary studies

Finnish survey

The first observational study of the relationship between dietary intake of antioxidant vitamins and subsequent coronary heart disease was a 14-year follow-up in more than 5,133 healthy men and women in Finland.[13] Food consumption, including intakes of dietary carotene, vitamin C and vitamin E, was estimated by dietary history, covering the total diet during the previous year.

An inverse association was observed between the dietary intake of vitamin E and coronary heart disease death rates in both men and women: those with higher intakes of vitamin E had lower death rates from coronary heart disease. The relative risks were 0.68 for men (P = 0.01) and 0.35 for women (P = <0.01), between the highest and lowest tertiles of intake. Similar associations were found for the dietary intake of vitamin C and carotenoids among women, and for the intake of important sources of those micronutrients, ie vegetables and fruit, among both men and women. These associations could not be attributed to confounding by any of the major non-dietary risk factors for coronary heart disease.

The authors conclude that, while their results support the hypothesis that antioxidant vitamins protect against coronary heart disease, the possibility that foods rich in these micronutrients may also contain other constituents that provide protection cannot be excluded.

The EURAMIC study

In the EURAMIC study,[14] an observational survey conducted in 10 centres in Europe, patients were recruited from coronary care units after their first myocardial infarction; controls for this study were subjects without a history of infarction. Results of this study showed a significant inverse relationship between beta-carotene levels in adipose tissue and the development of first myocardial infarction in nearly 1,500 previously healthy men. The relative risk of myocardial infarction in the lowest quintile of beta-carotene was 2.62 (odds ratio). The multivariate risk, taking into account other risk factors, was 1.78 (P = <0.001). There was no relationship between vitamin E (alpha-tocopherol) levels and risk of myocardial infarction. However, considering vitamin E (alpha-tocopherol) and beta-carotene together strengthened the relationship between the antioxidant vitamins and risk of myocardial infarction. In this study, both beta-carotene and vitamin E (alpha-tocopherol) were negatively associated with cigarette smoking. (For more information on the EURAMIC study, see Chapter 4.)

The Iowa Women's Health Study

The Iowa Women's Health Study,[15] a prospective cohort study of more than 34,000 postmenopausal women aged 55-69 years, examined the effect of intake of antioxidant vitamins on death rates from coronary heart disease. The study assessed the effect of consumption of antioxidant vitamins A, C and E both from food sources and from supplements. These were assessed using a dietary questionnaire, similar to that used in the Nurses Health Study[16] (see next page). Follow-up lasted seven years. The results were also adjusted to take into account smoking habits, physical inactivity, body mass index, total energy intake, alcohol intake, oestrogen replacement therapy, hypertension and diabetes mellitus.

Overall vitamin E consumption was inversely associated with death rates from coronary heart disease: a higher risk of coronary heart disease was associated with a lower level of vitamin E intake. However, the inverse association was for vitamin E derived from food, but not for vitamin E supplements. It remained significant, although weaker, when the other risk factors were taken into account. Attempts to identify vitamin E-rich foods which might have been responsible were unsuccessful. Intake of vitamins A and C and of retinol and carotenoids did not appear to be associated with the risk of death from coronary heart disease.

Studies of vitamin supplementation
Both the US Nurses' Health Study and a study of male health professionals in the US have looked at the effects of vitamin supplements on rates of coronary heart disease.

The US Nurses' Health Study of more than 87,000 women aged 34-59 suggests that, among middle-aged women, the use of vitamin E supplements may be associated with a reduced incidence of coronary heart disease, although interpretation of the results is difficult.[16] This study was conducted through postal dietary questionnaires and it also recorded multivitamin intake. The follow-up lasted up to eight years. The relative risk of major coronary disease was 0.54 and of death from cardiovascular disease was 0.58 among those taking vitamin E supplements, and 0.88 and 0.77 respectively among those taking multivitamins. Cautious interpretation is needed, since only 15% of the nurses took vitamin E and, of these, there were fewer current smokers, more who took vigorous activity and more taking hormone replacement therapy. This suggests that those taking vitamin E supplements were more health conscious and perhaps more healthy.

Another study[17] conducted in the US of nearly 40,000 male health professionals aged 40-75, had a similar design, based on a dietary questionnaire which assessed vitamin intakes from food sources and from supplements. The study found a lower risk of coronary heart disease in men with higher intakes of vitamin E. However, this association was weak when only dietary sources of vitamin E were taken into account; at the higher levels achieved with supplementation, the association became significant. Overall, for fatal coronary disease or non-fatal myocardial infarction, the multivariate relative risk between the highest and lowest quintiles for vitamin E intake was 0.63 (P<0.001). Among men who took vitamin E supplements of 100 IU or more a day for at least two years, the relative risk of coronary heart disease was less than for those who took lower supplements and for those who did not take such supplements.

The apparent protection was evident throughout the 10-year follow-up and was most significant in current smokers. The authors conclude that the association is weak and that it is not possible to rule out confounding, as in the Nurses' Health Study (ie those men with a higher intake of vitamin had healthier risk profiles). In this study, there was no association between the incidence of coronary heart disease and beta-carotene or vitamin C intakes.

Controlled trials

Over the last three years, several controlled trials of vitamin supplements have been published.

A randomised double-blind primary prevention trial was conducted in Finland among more than 29,000 male smokers aged 50-69, with a follow-up from five to eight years.[18] Participants took vitamin E, or beta-carotene, or both: the daily dose of vitamin E was 50mg, and that of beta-carotene 20mg. The primary aim was to determine the effects of these supplements on the incidence of lung cancer – which was not reduced – but the study also recorded death rates from coronary heart disease.

There was no difference in death rates from coronary heart disease between those taking vitamin E and the control group (rate per 10,000 person years in the vitamin E group = 71.0, compared to the rate in the control group of 75.0). There were more deaths from coronary heart disease in those who took beta-carotene supplements (mortality rate = 77.1) compared with the control group (68.9). The authors comment that an explanation for the lack of effect of these supplements on the incidence of lung cancer and coronary heart disease might be the low concentrations of vitamins used. However, the concentrations were sufficient to lead to a 40% increase in serum vitamin E (alpha-tocopherol) and a 1500% increase in beta-carotene concentrations after three years.

The findings of the Finnish trial have received support from an American multicentre, double-blind, randomised primary prevention trial (CARET)[19] in which the effects of a combination of 30mg beta-carotene and 25,000 IU of retinol (vitamin A) were studied in 18,300 smokers, former smokers and asbestos workers. After four years of supplementation, there was an increased risk of both cardiovascular disease (relative risk = 1.26) and of lung cancer (relative risk = 1.28). For these reasons, the trial was stopped 21 months prematurely.

The US Physicians Health Study[20] also investigated the effect of beta-carotene supplements in a well nourished population with low rates of coronary heart disease and cancer, using a randomised double-blind placebo controlled trial. The 22,000 male physicians who took part in this trial were allocated to one of four therapies:

- beta-carotene 50mg + aspirin 325mg on alternate days
- beta-carotene 50mg on alternate days + aspirin placebo
- aspirin 325mg on alternate days + beta-carotene placebo, or
- both placebos.

The follow-up was for 12 years. There were no differences in the incidence of cardiovascular diseases or cancer, or deaths from all causes.

A secondary prevention controlled trial, the Cambridge Heart Antioxidant Study (CHAOS),[21] examined the effect of vitamin E supplementation or placebo, on the risk of myocardial infarction in 2,002 patients with coronary atherosclerosis confirmed by angiography. The average follow-up time was 510 days. The effects of supplements of vitamin E capsules containing 400-800 IU were compared with those of placebo capsules of soybean oil. Among the treated group, plasma concentrations of vitamin E (alpha-tocopherol) nearly doubled. There were significantly fewer non-fatal myocardial infarctions (14 v 41 P<0.0001) in the vitamin E treated group, but there was an adverse trend for cardiovascular deaths. The only plasma lipid measured was total cholesterol, which did not change. However, this trial is unsatisfactory from several points of view: it was numerically small and therefore under-powered. It was stopped prematurely, and there appears to have been no review committee to classify cardiac events.

These trials are summarised in Table 3. As can be seen, none reduced the mortality from coronary heart disease and indeed beta-carotene may have increased it.

Table 3 *Four trials of antioxidant supplements in the prevention of coronary heart disease*

Trial	Numbers (antioxidants group and controls combined)	Age (years)	Follow-up (years)	Antioxidant	Relative risk of death from coronary heart disease (odds ratio)
PRIMARY PREVENTION					
Finnish Smokers[18]	14,564	50-69	5-8	vitamin E 50mg/day	0.94
	14,560	50-69	5-8	beta-carotene 20mg/day	1.12*
CARET (smokers)[19]	18,314	45-69	4	beta-carotene 30mg/day + 25,000 IU retinol	1.26*
US Physicians[20]	22,071	40-80	11	beta-carotene 50mg/2 days	1.09
SECONDARY PREVENTION					
CHAOS[21]	2,002	>55	<2	vitamin E 800-400mg/day	1.18**

* Overall mortality higher (P=0.02)
** Non-fatal myocardial infarction lower: odds ratio = 0.23 (P=0.005)

Conclusions

The scientific basis and rationale for increasing the intakes of vitamin E and C, and possibly beta-carotene, to reduce free radical attack and peroxidation of unstable lipoproteins is sound. It is hypothesised that oxidation of low density lipoprotein promotes atherosclerosis, leading to coronary heart disease, and that a high intake of antioxidant vitamins should reduce this risk.

Both the epidemiological evidence and that of observational studies indicate that there is an inverse relationship between dietary vitamin E intake and coronary heart disease mortality: higher intakes of dietary vitamin E are associated with lower death rates from coronary heart disease. All these studies showed that people who eat a relatively large quantity of vegetables, fruits and grains have low rates of cardiovascular disease. This may be due to high intakes of antioxidant vitamins or to 'the myriad of other substances in plants'[22] which might be protective, and which need to be examined for preventive properties.

While low plasma concentrations of vitamin E (alpha-tocopherol), and to a lesser extent of vitamin C, are found in patients with angina or myocardial infarction, the controlled clinical trials conducted so far do not provide sufficient sound evidence to conclude that supplements of vitamin E are beneficial. These trials have clearly indicated that there is no protection from coronary heart disease as a result of taking supplements of beta-carotene or vitamin A.

Further large-scale and long-term randomised controlled trials of the benefits of supplements of vitamin E, and also vitamin C, are needed.

Until then, it is not appropriate to recommend vitamin supplements as a means of protecting against coronary heart disease. The best possible advice is to eat more vegetables (the main source of vitamin E), cereals or olive oil, and fruit (the main source of vitamin C), particularly citrus fruit.

Public health advice along these lines needs more emphasis in populations with a high incidence of coronary disease with special focus on cigarette smokers. Much more interaction with the agricultural and retailing industries is needed in order to improve the availability and reduce the prices of these foods.

References

1   Diplock AT. Anti-oxidants and disease prevention. In: Baum H (ed). 1994. *Molecular Aspects of Medicine*. Elsevier Science; 15: 295-376.

2   Witztum JL. 1994. The oxidation hypothesis of atherosclerosis. *Lancet*; 344: 793-798.

3   Esterbauer H, Striegl G, Puhl H et al. 1989. The role of vitamin E and carotenoids in preventing oxidation of low-density lipoproteins. *Ann NY Acad Sci*; 570: 253-267.

4   Salonen JT, Salonen R, Seppanen K, Rinta-Kiika S et al. 1991. Effects of anti-oxidant supplementation on platelet function: a randomized pair-matched, placebo-controlled, double-blind trial in men with low anti-oxidant status. *American Journal of Clinical Nutrition*; 53: 1222-1229.

5   Verlangieri AJ, Bush MJ. 1992. Effects of d-a-tocopherol supplementation on experimentally induced primate atherosclerosis. *Journal of the American College of Nutrition*; 11: 131-138.

6   Riemersma RA, Oliver MF, Elton RA et al. 1990. Plasma antioxidants and coronary heart disease: vitamins C and E and selenium. *European Journal of Clinical Nutrition*; 44: 143-150.

7   Gey KF, Puska P, Jordan P, Moser UK. 1991. Inverse correlation between plasma vitamin E and mortality from ischemic heart disease in cross-cultural epidemiology. *American Journal of Clinical Nutrition*; 53: 326-334.

8   Gregory J, Foster K, Tyler H, Wiseman M for the Office of Population Censuses and Surveys. 1990. *The Dietary and Nutritional Survey of British Adults*. London: HMSO.

9   Fulton M, Thomson M, Elton RA et al. 1988. Cigarette smoking, social class and nutrient intake: relevance to coronary heart disease. *European Journal of Clinical Nutrition*; 42: 797-803.

10 Frankel EN, Kanner J, German GB et al. 1993. Inhibition of oxidation of human low-density lipoprotein by phenolic substances in red wine. *Lancet*; 341: 454-457.

11 Bolton-Smith C, Smith WCS, Woodward M, Tunstall-Pedoe H. 1991. Nutrient intakes of different social-class groups: results from the Scottish Heart Health Study (SHHS). *British Journal of Nutrition*; 65: 321-335.

12 Riemersma RA, Wood DA, Macintyre CAA et al. 1991. Risk of angina pectoris and plasma concentrations of vitamins A, C and E and carotene. *Lancet*; 337: 1-5.

13 Knekt P, Reunanen A, Järvinen R et al. 1994. Antioxidant vitamin intake and coronary mortality in a longitudinal population. *American Journal of Epidemiology*; 139: 1180-1189.

14 Kardinaal AFM, Kok FJ, Gomez-Aracena J et al. 1993. Antioxidants in adipose tissue and risk of myocardial infarction: the EURAMIC study. *Lancet*; 342: 1379-1384.

15 Kushi LH, Folsom AR, Prineas RJ et al. 1996. Dietary antioxidants and death from coronary heart disease in postmenopausal women. *New England Journal of Medicine*; 334: 1156-1162.

16 Stampfer MK, Hennekens CH, Manson JE et al. 1993. Vitamin E consumption and the risk of coronary heart disease in women. *New England Journal of Medicine*; 328: 1444-1449.

17 Rimm EB, Stampfer MJ, Ascherio A et al. 1993. Vitamin E consumption and the risk of coronary heart disease in men. *New England Journal of Medicine*; 328: 1450-1456.

18 The Alpha-Tocopherol, Beta Carotene Cancer Prevention Study Group. 1994. The effect of vitamin E and beta carotene on the incidence of lung cancer and other cancers in male smokers. *New England Journal of Medicine*; 330: 1029-1035.

19 Omenn GS, Goodman GE, Thornquist MD et al. 1996. Effect of a combination of beta carotene and vitamin A on lung cancer and cardiovascular disease. *New England Journal of Medicine*; 334: 1150-1155.

20 Hennekens CH, Buring JE, Manson JE et al. 1996. Lack of effect of longterm supplementation with betacarotene on the incidence of malignant neoplasms and cardiovascular disease. *New England Journal of Medicine*; 334: 1145-1149.

21 Stephens NG, Parsons A, Schofield PM et al. 1996. Randomised controlled trial of vitamin E in patients with coronary disease: Cambridge Heart Antioxidant Study (CHAOS). *Lancet*; 347: 781-786.

22 Greenberg ER, Sporn MB. 1996. Antioxidant vitamins, cancer, and cardiovascular disease. *New England Journal of Medicine*; 334: 1189-1190.

Professor Michael Oliver CBE is an individual member of the National Heart Forum, and is Professor Emeritus, University of Edinburgh.

Chapter 3

Do vegetables and fruit protect against coronary heart disease? Studies among vegetarians

Dr Margaret Thorogood

Health Promotion Sciences Unit, London School of Hygiene and Tropical Medicine

Introduction

A number of studies of people who eat a diet rich in fruit and vegetables, and therefore rich in antioxidant nutrients, have tried to test the hypothesis that fruit and vegetables lower the risk of coronary heart disease. Vegetarians generally have high intakes of cereals, nuts and vegetable oils, carrots and green vegetables as well as fruit. Such a diet is rich in vitamins E, C and beta-carotene. (See Appendix for information on foods rich in these vitamins.) However, vegetarians differ from the rest of the population in a number of important ways: they tend to smoke less, have lower body mass index (BMI) and lower alcohol intakes, and come predominantly from social classes I and II - all of which are known to confer a health advantage. It has proved difficult to disentangle these different effects.

This chapter summarises the findings of studies of vegetarians in Oxford and in Germany, users of 'health food' shops in the UK, and studies of Seventh Day Adventists, who for religious reasons abstain from tobacco and alcohol and many of whom follow a vegetarian diet.

The Oxford Vegetarian Study

The Oxford Vegetarian Study was set up to test the idea that people eating a vegetarian diet may experience lower rates of certain cancers and coronary heart disease. Between 1980 and 1984 some 6,115 non meat eaters* were recruited to the study through advertising in the press, including publications of the Vegetarian Society of the UK.

---

*   Non meat eaters fell into three groups. Vegetarians were defined as people who did not eat meat or fish or ate these foods less than once a week. They ate eggs and/or dairy products. Vegans did not eat meat, fish, eggs or dairy products. Fish eaters did not eat meat or ate meat less than once a week, may or may not have eaten eggs or dairy products, and ate fish at least once a week.

The vegetarians were asked to nominate their meat-eating friends and relatives to take part in the study. In this way, 5,015 meat eaters were recruited to the study to serve as controls. By using this method of selecting participants, the study and control groups were similar in terms of their social class, interest in health and attitudes to exercise. They differed in smoking habit, with the vegetarians tending to smoke less. Both the vegetarians and the control group smoked less than the general population; smoking prevalence in the early 1980s was 34% compared with 23% in the control group and 15% in the vegetarian cohort. The vegetarians tended to have lower body mass index than the control group.

Study participants were asked to keep a four-day dietary record. Approximately half of all participants submitted completed records. Overall mortality rates, deaths from cancer and coronary heart disease were recorded.[1, 2] Follow-up continued until 1993.

Results

Diet

Analysis of a subsample of 200 dietary records showed that all the participants ate more fruit and vegetables, and substantially more grains, pasta and nuts than the general population. Cakes, puddings and biscuits were eaten in the same amounts as the general population, although these tended to be home-made with whole wheat flour and vegetable oils. The meat eater controls on average ate half as much meat as the general population. All participants in the study consumed less milk, eggs, fat, sugar, jam and potatoes than the general population. Very little hard margarine or ordinary soft margarine (not polyunsaturated margarines) were consumed.[1]

Deaths from all causes, coronary heart disease and cancer

Standardised mortality ratios (SMRs) for deaths from all causes, cancers and coronary heart disease were calculated for participants in the Oxford Vegetarian Study compared with the general population. Lower rates of coronary heart disease were seen in participants in the study (meat eaters and vegetarians) compared with the general population. Much of this difference was due to the lower rates of smoking, and higher social class of the study participants. When the SMRs for vegetarians were compared with the control group, the vegetarians had a lower rate of all cause mortality, and mortality from cancers and coronary heart disease (see Figure 1). When these figures were adjusted for the difference between the two groups for BMI, smoking and social class, the vegetarian death rate from all causes was 20% lower than in the controls.[2]

Among vegetarians the death rate from coronary heart disease was half that of the meat eaters (see Figure 1). However, when the figures were adjusted for BMI, smoking and social class, the difference in death rates from coronary heart disease was no longer significant.

An analysis of the death rates for coronary heart disease in those people – meat eaters and non meat eaters – who had never smoked, suggested that the vegetarians might be protected from coronary heart disease (see Table 1). The number of people studied was small and the confidence intervals larger, but the point estimates were similar. It is still not clear from these results whether the vegetarians had a lower rate of coronary heart disease because they did not eat meat, or because of their higher consumption of fruit and vegetables.

Figure 1 *Oxford Vegetarian Study: standardised mortality ratio by cause*

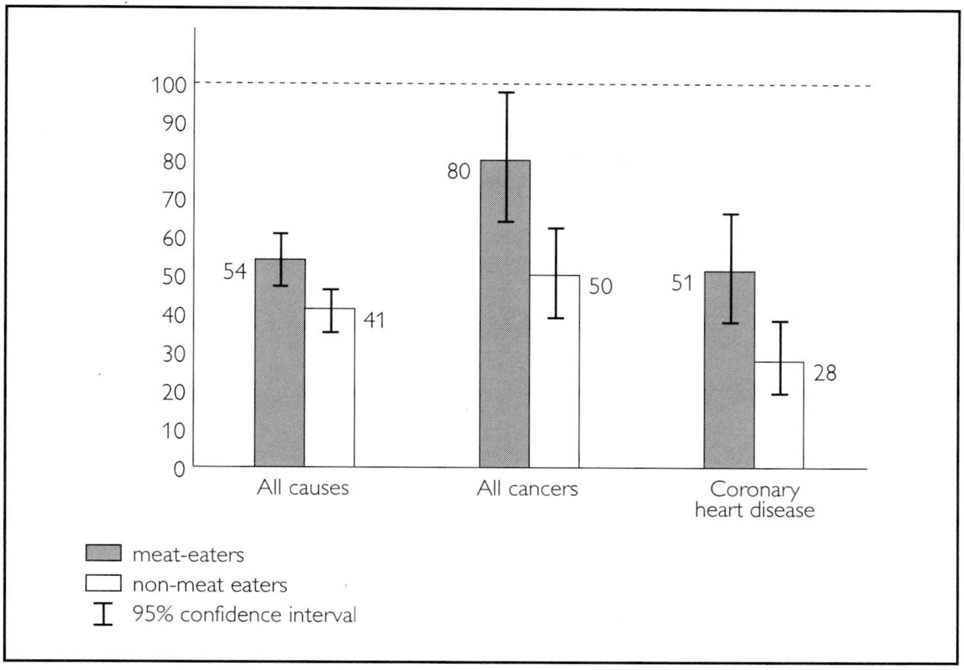

Source: See reference 2.

Table 1 *Adjusted death rate ratios for all cause and coronary heart disease mortality in vegetarians compared with controls, in the Oxford Vegetarian Study*

	Cause of death	
	All cause (95% confidence interval)	Coronary heart disease (95% confidence interval)
Unadjusted	0.75 (0.62, 0.91)	0.55 (0.36, 0.82)
Adjusted for body mass index, smoking, and social class	0.80 (0.65, 0.99)	0.72 (0.47, 1.10)
Never smokers		
Unadjusted	0.85 (0.62, 1.15)	0.54 (0.26, 1.09)
Adjusted for body mass index and social class	0.81 (0.59, 1.12)	0.59 (0.28, 1.24)

Source: See reference 2.

The Health Food Shop Users Study

Ten years before the Oxford Vegetarian Study was set up, some 11,000 people were recruited* for a study of the effect of a vegetarian diet on death rates from coronary heart disease.[3] Of the 11,000 people recruited, 43% were vegetarian, mostly lactoovovegetarians (vegetarians who eat eggs and/or dairy products). All participants were asked to fill in a brief screening questionnaire which included a question on vegetarianism. A subset of 300 people (meat eaters and vegetarians) was visited personally. More detailed dietary information was obtained and blood was collected for analysis of total and HDL cholesterol measurement. Blood pressure, height and weight were also measured.

Results

The results after 17 years showed that daily consumption of fresh fruit was associated with a 24% reduction in mortality from coronary heart disease, a 32% reduction in mortality from cerebrovascular disease, and a 21% reduction in all cause mortality compared with less frequent consumption.

All study participants had lower death rates from all causes than the general population. Data from the subset who were visited suggested that study participants tended to be non-smokers, of higher social class than the general population. The vegetarians had a lower mean BMI than the meat eaters. There was no consistent difference in blood pressure between the meat eaters and vegetarians.

Table 2 *Deaths from all causes, coronary heart disease and cerebrovascular disease in the Health Food Shop Users Study*

Cause of death	Adjusted mortality ratios (95% confidence interval)	
	Ate fresh fruit daily	Did not eat fresh fruit daily
All causes	0.79 (0.70, 0.90)*	1.0
Coronary heart disease	0.76 (0.60, 0.97)**	1.0
Cerebrovascular disease	0.68 (0.47, 0.98)**	1.0

* two tailed P<0.05
** P<0.01

Source: See reference 3.

---

* Participants in the study were recruited through the Holland and Barrett health food shop chain. In addition participants included members of the Vegan Society, Vegetarian Society, Jewish Vegetarian Society and the McCarrison Society and subscribers to the magazines *Here's Health, Health for All, Good Health* and *British Advent Messenger*.

The German Vegetarian Study

In 1978, a small study of 2,000 vegetarians and people 'leading a health conscious lifestyle' was set up in the Federal Republic of Germany, to explore the relationship between vegetarianism and coronary heart disease.[4] Study participants filled in a detailed questionnaire on diet, smoking, drinking, socioeconomic status and physical activity. The questionnaire also elicited information on fasting, meditation and family medical history. Death rates in the cohort of vegetarians were compared with deaths in the general population, rather than a control group, after 11 years' follow-up. The study participants were generally better educated and of higher socioeconomic status, with lower BMI and smoking rates than the general population.

The study cohort was subdivided into 'moderate' and 'strict' vegetarians. 'Moderate vegetarians' ate meat 'occasionally' (although it is not clear how often or how much meat was consumed). Sixty-one per cent (521 out of 858 men and 642 out of 1,046 women) of the cohort were in this category. 'Strict vegetarians' avoided meat and fish completely and comprised 39% of the cohort (337 men and 404 women).

Results

The cohort experienced about half the mortality rates of the general population (see Table 3). There was half the expected number of deaths from cardiovascular diseases. The largest reduction in mortality was for coronary heart disease where the observed mortality was one-third of that expected.

Table 3 *All cause and circulatory diseases mortality analysis from the German Vegetarian Study (1978-1989)*

Cause of death ICD 9th series	Standardised mortality ratios *(95% confidence interval)*	
	Men	Women
All causes ICD 001-999	0.44 *(0.36, 0.53)*	0.53 *(0.44, 0.64)*
Circulatory system ICD 390-459	0.39 *(0.29, 0.51)*	0.46 *(0.35, 0.60)*

Source: See reference 4.

Although the 'strict' vegetarians had a higher mortality overall than 'moderate' vegetarians, the mortality from coronary heart disease was lower (see Figure 2). These data suggest that some component of the vegetarian diet (not necessarily the avoidance of meat) may be protective against coronary heart disease.

Figure 2 *Relative risk of mortality in 'moderate' vs 'strict' vegetarianism in the German Vegetarian Study*

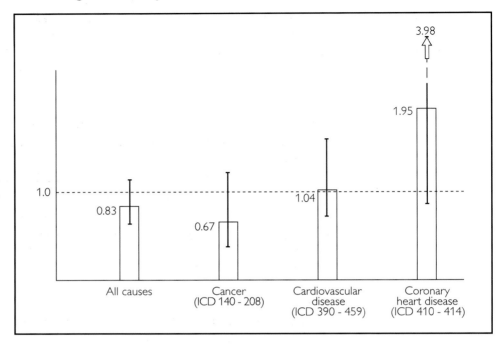

Source: See reference 4.

The effect of meat and non-meat diets on blood pressure

Several studies have suggested that a vegetarian diet protects against high blood pressure. A number of randomised trials, mainly in Australia, have been carried out which show that people who start to follow a vegetarian diet reduce their blood pressure.[5] The trial by Prescott et al, in 1988, put people onto two diets which it was believed would reduce blood pressure. In one diet 40% of the protein came from meat; in the other none of the protein came from meat.

Both diets were equally ineffective at lowering blood pressure (see Table 4). It made no difference whether the protein in the diet came from meat or not. This suggests that some element other than the absence of meat in the vegetarian diet acts to reduce blood pressure.

Table 4 *The effect on blood pressure of diets with different protein sources*

Sitting blood pressure (mmHg)	Difference in blood pressure *(95% confidence interval)*	
	Meat eaters (40% of protein from meat)	Non meat eaters (0% of protein from meat)
Systolic	−0.3 *(−2.5, +2.0)*	+2.2 *(−0.0, +4.4)*
Diastolic	+0.1 *(−1.9, +2.1)*	+0.9 *(−0.5, +2.2)*

Source: See reference 6.

Studies of Seventh Day Adventists

Much interesting data on mortality rates and diets rich in fruit and vegetables have come from long-term studies of Seventh Day Adventist religious communities. These communities are large and well organised with reliable registers of members. One large cohort in California has been studied since the 1960s.

Seventh Day Adventists abstain from tobacco and alcohol, and about half are vegetarian. Of the meat eaters none eat pork, and beef is the main meat consumed. Extensive dietary and lifestyle information has been obtained by questionnaire from the cohort, including a food frequency survey, history of hypertension, diabetes and coronary heart disease, height and weight data, smoking and exercise habits. In addition, the data on coronary heart disease mortality has been analysed according to the frequency of nut consumption.[7, 8] The control groups included people who did not belong to the Seventh Day Adventist community and who did not smoke.

Results

Standardised mortality ratios (SMRs) of Californian Adventists were compared with those of non-smoking men and women who had completed the same questionnaire (see Figure 3). In women, there was no difference between the Adventists and the non-smoking non-Adventists with respect to coronary heart disease, but there was a significantly lower SMR in men.

Figure 3 *Standardised mortality ratios of Adventists compared with non-smokers completing the same questionnaire*

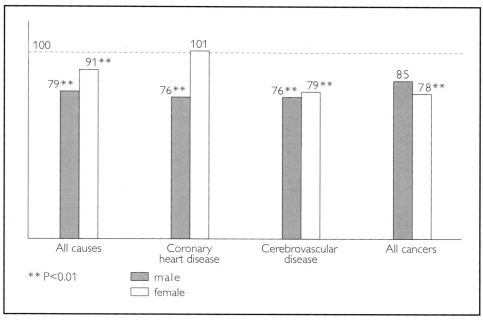

Source: See reference 7.

When the effect of eating beef on the relative risk of a fatal coronary heart disease event was calculated, it was found that, in men, the relative risk of a fatal coronary heart disease event increased markedly with the number of times beef was eaten each week. Men who ate beef three times a week had more than twice the rate of fatal coronary heart disease compared to those who never ate beef. In women, there was no relationship between frequency of beef consumption and the rate of fatal coronary heart disease.

Table 5   The effect of beef consumption on the risk of a fatal coronary heart disease event: results from the Californian Adventist Study

Frequency of beef consumption	Relative risk of a fatal coronary heart disease event *(95% confidence interval)*	
	Men	Women
Never	1.0	1.0
< three times a week	1.9 *(1.1, 3.3)*	0.8 *(0.5, 1.3)*
≥ three times a week	2.3 *(1.1, 4.8)*	0.8 *(0.4, 1.6)*

Source: See reference 8.

These data may suggest that, in men, avoiding meat rather than choosing fruit and vegetables was the important factor in lowering the risk of coronary heart disease.

Figure 4   Relative risk of coronary heart disease events by nut consumption in the Californian Adventist Study

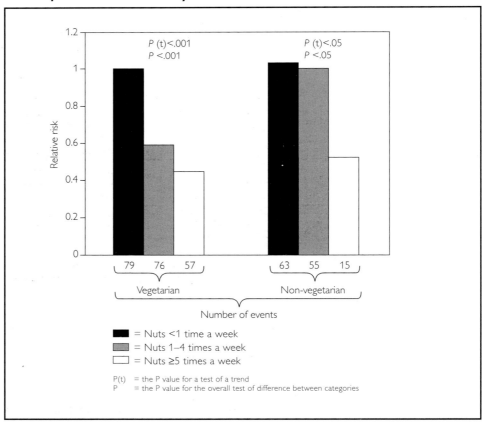

Source: See reference 8.

Preventing coronary heart disease. The role of antioxidants, vegetables and fruit

The study also examined the relative risk of coronary heart disease according to the frequency of nut consumption. Participants in the study were divided into three groups: regular nut consumers; people who consumed nuts one to three times each week; and people who did not eat nuts. The risk of coronary heart disease events reduced as nut intake increased (see Figure 4). These data suggest that, if this relationship is causal, it is the vitamin E content of the nuts or the polyunsaturated fat content of the diet which lowers the risk of coronary heart disease. However, it was not possible to separate out these two effects from these data.[9]

Conclusion

It is always difficult to establish relationships between intake of individual foods or nutrients and coronary heart disease in epidemiologic studies. All diets consist of a complex combination of foods. A diet that has no meat, for example, is likely to be a diet with a high proportion of fruit and vegetables, and it is difficult to determine which aspect of the diet is offering an observed health benefit. Even when a particular food can be isolated, as in the case of nut intake, it is not possible to be sure which of the nutrients contained in that food is or are the important factors.

In summary, although the observational studies of vegetarians and diets rich in fruit and vegetables (and antioxidant nutrients) cannot provide conclusive evidence, they do support the hypothesis that such a diet might lower the risk of coronary heart disease.

References

1　Thorogood M, Roe L, McPherson K, Mann J. 1990. Dietary intake and plasma lipid levels: lessons from a study of the diet of health conscious groups. *British Medical Journal;* 300: 1297-1301.

2　Thorogood M, Mann J, Appleby P, McPherson K. 1994. Risk of death from cancer and ischaemic heart disease in meat and non-meat eaters. *British Medical Journal;* 308: 1667-1671.

3　Key T, Thorogood M, Appleby P, Burr M. 1996. Dietary habits and mortality in 11,000 vegetarians and health conscious people: results of a 17 year follow up. *British Medical Journal;* 313: 775-779.

4　Chang-Claude J, Frentzel-Beyme R, Eilber U. 1992. Mortality pattern of German vegetarians after 11 years of follow-up. *Epidemiology;* 3 (5): 395-401.

5　Thorogood M. 1995. Epidemiology of vegetarianism and health. *Nutrition Research Reviews;* 8: 179-192.

6　Prescott SL, Jenner DA, Beilin LJ, Margetts BM, Vongongen R. 1988. A randomized controlled trial of the effect on blood pressure of dietary non-meat protein versus meat protein in normotensive omnivores. *Clinical Science;* 74: 665-672.

7　Phillips RL, Kuzma JW, Beeson WL, Lotz T. 1980. Influence of selection versus lifestyle on risk of fatal cancer and cardiovascular disease among Seventh-Day Adventists. *American Journal of Epidemiology;* 112 (2): 296-314.

8　Fraser GE, Sabaté J, Beeson WL, Strahan TM. 1992. A possible protective effect of nut consumption on risk of coronary heart disease: The Adventist Health Study. *Archives of Internal Medicine;* 152: 1416-1424.

9　Fraser GE, Beeson WL, Phillips RL. 1991. Diet and lung cancer in California Seventh-day Adventists. *American Journal of Epidemiology;* 133 (7): 683-693.

Chapter 4

Antioxidant nutrients and coronary heart disease: international evidence from the EURAMIC study

Professor Frans Kok

Department of Epidemiology and Public Health, Wageningen Agricultural University, Netherlands

Introduction

The EURAMIC study (European Antioxidant Myocardial Infarction and Cancer of the Breast), is an international case control study.* One of its aims is to examine the relationship between tissue levels of a number of antioxidant biomarkers, such as vitamin E and beta-carotene, and the risk of myocardial infarction in people in 10 study centres in Europe, including Scotland. The EURAMIC study examined only certain antioxidant nutrients. In common with many other studies, it did not look directly at intakes of fruits and vegetables, which contain a number and range of different bioactive compounds.[1, 2, 3]

In 1995, the Dutch Board of Fruits and Vegetables commissioned a group of epidemiologists, scientists and clinicians, many of whom are involved in the EURAMIC study, to prepare a report on the evidence of the role fruit and vegetables play in relation to chronic diseases.[4] This report formed the rationale and basis for a public promotion campaign. An examination of all the evidence from epidemiological studies revealed that information relating coronary heart disease directly to fruits and vegetables was lacking. Information on the role of fruit and vegetables with respect to cancer is more readily available, and recommendations to increase fruit and vegetable consumption to at least 400g a day, or at least five portions a day, are based predominantly on evidence from these studies.

---

*   The EURAMIC study involved multi-disciplinary teams of scientists, clinicians and epidemiologists in Finland (Helsinki), Germany (Berlin), Israel (Jerusalem), Netherlands (Zeist), Norway (Sarpsborg), Russia (Moscow), Spain (Granada and Malaga), Switzerland (Zurich), and the UK (Scotland). The coordination of the study was sponsored under the European Union BIOMED programme.

The major dietary sources of antioxidant nutrients

Table 1 shows the major dietary sources of antioxidant nutrients, vitamins C, E and beta-carotene, in the Netherlands, and the recommended dietary allowances. (See also the Appendix.) Although fruit and vegetables are rich sources of a wide variety of antioxidant nutrients, other products, such as margarines and oils, are a major source of dietary vitamin E. In the Netherlands and many other European countries, the intake of vitamins E and C and beta-carotene seems to be sufficient to prevent nutrient deficiencies. However, the question remains as to whether current intakes are optimal to prevent chronic diseases.

Table 1 *Major dietary sources of antioxidants in the Netherlands and recommended dietary allowances*

Nutrient	Major dietary sources	Recommended dietary allowances	
		Men (mg)	Women (mg)
Vitamin E	Vegetable oils and fats, margarines, nuts, fish	7-8	6-6.5
Vitamin C	Fruits and vegetables, potatoes	60	60
Beta-carotene	Green-yellow and leafy vegetables	6*	4.8*

* Based on the retinol equivalent

The EURAMIC study: design

The EURAMIC study examined a range of biomarkers in the adipose tissue in male patients with a first myocardial infarction, admitted to the coronary care unit within 24 hours after the onset of the first symptoms. The levels of selected fat soluble antioxidants were compared with those of population controls or hospital patients from the same catchment area, who had no previous history of myocardial infarction or coronary heart disease. Only men under 70 years of age were studied; women were not included in the study.

Individuals included in the study had to have a stable diet in the past year, with no weight change of more than 5kg over the same period. Very few people in the study took dietary supplements. Those who did had to have had stable supplement use. Data from 683 cases and 727 controls were analysed. Past intakes of fruits and vegetables were not measured, because this could not be done accurately. The levels of a spectrum of fatty acids in adipose tissue, including trans-fatty acids, were also analysed. This enabled the antioxidant nutrient content in the adipose tissue to be related to the total level of fatty acid in the adipose tissue.

In addition, traditional risk factors for coronary heart disease such as smoking, hypertension, cholesterol levels, diabetes, family history, alcohol intake and body mass index (BMI) were examined in patients and controls. This enabled any effect of antioxidant nutrients on the risk of myocardial infarction to be disentangled from the effect of traditional risk factors for coronary heart disease.

Results of the EURAMIC study

Traditional coronary heart disease risk factor profiles

Traditional coronary heart disease risk factors such as hypertension, smoking and BMI were significantly higher in myocardial infarction patients than controls. The incidence of diabetes was about the same. Family history and alcohol use were slightly lower in controls, but this was not significant. The measurement of cholesterol levels was not very reliable in cases in the acute phase of myocardial infarction. Nevertheless, cholesterol levels were lower in myocardial infarction patients than in controls (although this was only just statistically significant; see Table 2). The results for these risk factors in myocardial infarction patients compared with controls match the results of previous studies and give credibility and validity to the results of the study.

Table 2 *Risk factors for myocardial infarction in the EURAMIC study*

Risk factor	Number of cases (683)	Number of controls (727)	Difference*	(95% confidence interval)
Age (years)	54.7	53.3	1.5	(0.6, 2.4)
Total cholesterol (mmol/l)	5.4	5.6	- 0.2	(0.3, 0)
Hypertension (%)	26	17	12	(7, 17)
Smoking (%)	56	33	29	(24, 34)
Diabetes (%)	8	4	3	(2, 4)
Family history of coronary heart disease (%)	57	43	13	(8, 19)
Alcohol use (%)	80	82	-1	(-4, 3)
BMI (kg/m^2)	26.5	26	0.5	(0.1, 0.9)

* Adjusted for age and study centre

Source: See reference 1.

Antioxidant nutrient levels in myocardial infarction patients and controls

Table 3 shows the tissue levels of vitamin E and beta-carotene in myocardial infarction patients and controls. There was no difference in the mean level of adipose vitamin E in the myocardial infarction cases compared with the controls. However, the level of beta-carotene was 17% lower in myocardial infarction cases than in controls. This mean difference of 0.07µg/g was statistically significant, when the figures were adjusted for age and centre (95% confidence interval 0.04, 0.1).

Table 3 Tissue levels of vitamin E and beta-carotene

Antioxidant nutrient	Tissue levels (µg/g)	
	Myocardial infarction patients	Controls
Vitamin E	193	192
Beta-carotene	0.35	0.42

Source: See reference 1.

Antioxidant nutrients, traditional risk factors and myocardial infarction

The relationship between vitamin concentrations in the adipose tissue and risk factors for coronary heart disease was measured in the controls. There was an inverse association between the levels of beta-carotene or vitamin E and the number of cigarettes smoked per day.* In other words, the more cigarettes smoked each day, the lower the levels of beta-carotene or vitamin E measured in the adipose tissue. The same relationship was observed between beta-carotene or vitamin E levels and BMI.† Individuals with the lowest BMI had the highest levels of beta-carotene or vitamin E. People with a family history of coronary heart disease had significantly higher beta-carotene levels,‡ and also higher levels of HDL cholesterol.§ There was no significant correlation between tissue levels of vitamin E or beta-carotene and the other risk factors measured, namely age, serum cholesterol, alcohol use, angina pectoris, diabetes, or history of hypertension.

No association was found between vitamin E level and risk of myocardial infarction, when the data were adjusted for age, smoking, BMI (a crude indication of energy intake and expenditure) or study centre (see Table 4).

Table 4 Risk of myocardial infarction for quintiles of vitamin E

	Quintiles of vitamin E				
	Lowest	2	3	4	Highest
Median (µg/g)	103	149	198	253	385
Number of myocardial infarction cases	136	132	136	144	135
Number of controls	146	146	145	145	146
Simple odds ratio*	0.9	0.9	1	1.1	1
Multivariate odds ratio**	0.8	0.9	1	1.1	1

* Adjusted for age and centre
** Adjusted for age, centre, smoking and BMI

Source: See reference 1.

---

*   (beta-carotene: r = -0.15, p<0.05; vitamin E: r = -0.13, p = 0.053)
†   (beta-carotene: r = -0.35, p<0.001; vitamin E: r = -0.12, p = 0.001)
‡   (r = 0.01, p = 0.08)
§   (r = 0.28, p<0.001)

Preventing coronary heart disease. The role of antioxidants, vegetables and fruit

When the data for levels of beta-carotene were analysed in the same way, it was found that people with the lowest levels of beta-carotene had an increased risk of acute myocardial infarction (see Table 5). The simple odds ratio for individuals with beta-carotene levels in the lowest quintile was 2.6, or 1.8 after adjustment for age, study centre, smoking and BMI.

Table 5 *Risk of myocardial infarction for quintiles of beta-carotene*

| | Quintiles of beta-carotene | | | | |
	Lowest	2	3	4	Highest
Median (µg/g)	0.15	0.3	0.45	0.65	1.11
Number of myocardial infarction cases	177	184	124	119	79
Number of controls	145	146	145	145	146
Simple odds ratio*	2.6	2.5	1.7	1.5	1.0
Multivariate odds ratio**	1.8	1.8	1.4	1.3	1.0
95% confidence interval	(1.2, 2.7)	(1.2, 2.6)	(0.9, 2.1)	(0.9, 1.9)	

* Adjusted for age and centre
** Adjusted for age, centre, smoking and BMI

Source: See reference 1.

There was also a graded association between levels of beta-carotene and risk of myocardial infarction according to smoking status. There was an inverse association between low levels of beta-carotene and myocardial infarction in current and ex-smokers. Figure 1 shows the risk of myocardial infarction in the

Figure 1 *Risk of myocardial infarction for beta-carotene according to smoking*

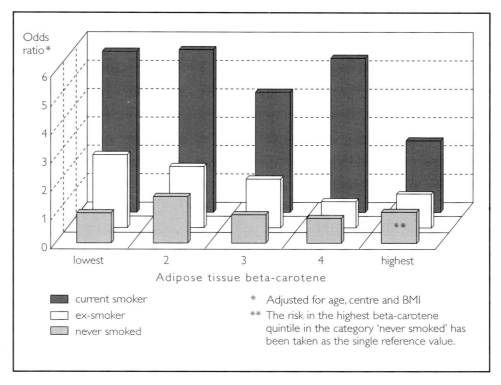

Source: See reference 1.

quintiles of the beta-carotene distribution, but also takes into account the higher risk conferred by smoking. In those in the highest beta-carotene quintile, the risk of myocardial infarction for ex-smokers as compared with people who had never smoked was 1.22 (odds ratio), whereas it was 2.34 for current smokers.

Conclusions

The EURAMIC study results do not suggest an important role for vitamin E in lowering the risk of coronary heart disease, at levels achieved through the diet. This is in line with other observational epidemiological studies such as the findings from two large US prospective studies in female nurses and male health professionals.[5, 6] In the Nurses Study[5] a 41% reduction in coronary heart disease risk was seen only among those who used vitamin E supplements. Those people with lower intakes of vitamin E, within the normal dietary range, had a lower risk of coronary heart disease of 0.79. However, this was not statistically significant. In the study of male health professionals[6] a comparable reduction in risk of coronary heart disease of 36% was seen only in those men with very high intakes of vitamin E achieved through supplement use. In both these studies, when the cohorts were subdivided into quintiles by vitamin E consumption, a 40% reduction in coronary heart disease risk was seen only in those subjects taking supplements, ie mega-doses of vitamin E (see Chapter 2).

The exception may be in populations, such as in Scotland, where very low levels of vitamin E appear to be associated with an increased risk of myocardial infarction.[7] Data from the Scottish centre in the EURAMIC study support this conclusion. However, these results alone do not justify making quantitative recommendations for vitamin E intakes. Any potential benefit of vitamin E supplements needs to await the results of randomised controlled trials.

The EURAMIC study showed that very low levels of beta-carotene were associated with an increased risk of myocardial infarction. Epidemiological evidence suggests that the benefits of high levels of beta-carotene from dietary sources may be limited to current and ex-smokers. This is consistent with the results from the US prospective studies. In these studies a protective effect was also seen most clearly in people who were current smokers. An overall 25% reduction in risk of coronary heart disease was observed in people with dietary intakes of beta-carotene in the highest quintiles. The results of trials of beta-carotene supplements in current smokers point to the need for caution, with increased rates of cardiovascular disease, lung cancer and overall mortality in these individuals.[8]* Dietary advice for current and ex-smokers should stress the need to increase the consumption of fruits and vegetables.

No association between vitamin C intake and risk of coronary heart disease was seen in the US prospective studies.

---

* The CARET (Beta-Carotene and Retinol Efficacy Trial) of beta-carotene at 30mg/day in 17,700 male and female smokers, and male smokers with asbestos exposure, was terminated 21 months early, due to the excess of deaths from lung cancer and all cause mortality, in those individuals taking beta-carotene supplements. *Lancet* 1996; 347: 249.

Preventing coronary heart disease. The role of antioxidants, vegetables and fruit

The US prospective studies may have examined a specific population of supplement users who differ in many aspects from the general population. However, the data from the EURAMIC study, which examined a more general population, are in line with the results from these cohort studies.

Over the last five years in the Netherlands fruit and vegetable intakes have been decreasing. The decrease has been an average of 10% over this time and is especially marked in younger age groups.[9] The current average consumption level of 242g of fruits and vegetables per day is similar to that reported in the UK. This is particularly worrying since atherosclerosis is a long pathological process and therefore campaigns are needed to reverse these trends in the under-50-year-olds. A campaign to increase fruit and vegetable consumption in the Netherlands is already under way. The results from the EURAMIC study suggest that recommendations on the use of antioxidant nutrient supplements should await well-designed clinical trials.

References

1   Kardinaal AFM, Kok FJ, Ringstad J et al. 1993. Antioxidants in adipose tissue and risk of myocardial infarction: the EURAMIC study. *Lancet*; 342: 1379-1384.

2   Kardinaal AFM, Aro A, Kark JD et al. 1995. Association between beta-carotene and acute myocardial infarction depends on poly-unsaturated fatty acid status: The EURAMIC study. *Arteriosclerosis, Thrombosis and Vascular Biology*; 15: 726-732.

3   Kardinaal AFM, Van't Veer P, Brants HAM et al. 1995. Relations between antioxidant vitamins in adipose tissue, plasma and diet. *American Journal of Epidemiology*; 141: 440-450.

4   Jansen MCJF, Van't Veer P, Kok FJ. 1995. *Fruits and Vegetables in Chronic Disease Prevention: Rationale for Fruits and Vegetables Campaign*. Wageningen, Netherlands: Department of Epidemiology and Public Health, Wageningen Agricultural University.

5   Stampfer MJ, Hennekens CH, Manson JE et al. 1993. Vitamin E consumption and risk of coronary disease in women. *New England Journal of Medicine*; 328: 1444-1449.

6   Rimm EB, Stampfer MJ, Ascherio A et al. 1993. Vitamin E consumption and the risk of coronary heart disease in men. *New England Journal of Medicine*; 328: 1450-1456.

7   Riemersma RA, Wood DA, Macintyre CCA et al. 1991. Risk of angina pectoris and plasma concentrations of vitamins A, C and E and carotene. *Lancet*; 337: 1-5.

8   The Alpha Tocopherol, Beta Carotene Cancer Prevention Study Group. 1994. The effect of vitamin E and Beta carotene on the incidence of lung cancer and other cancers in male smokers. *New England Journal of Medicine*; 330: 1029-1035.

9   Dutch Board of Fruits and Vegetables. 1994. *Consumption of Vegetables, Fruits, Nuts and Fruit Juices in the Netherlands. National Nutrition Survey 1992*. (In Dutch.) The Hague, Netherlands: Dutch Board of Fruits and Vegetables.

Part 4

Dietary recommendations on vegetables and fruit

Changing rationales, consistent advice: dietary recommendations on vegetables and fruit

Carol Williams

Nutrition Consultant

Professor Michael Marmot

Department of Epidemiology and Public Health, University College London

Introduction

There is a considerable and growing body of evidence which suggests that diets rich in vegetables and fruit, and the antioxidant nutrients they contain, are protective against a wide range of chronic diseases and degenerative conditions associated with ageing.[1, 2, 3] These include coronary heart disease, many cancers and cataracts.

Healthy eating advice to the public encouraging increased consumption of fruit and vegetables has remained remarkably consistent over the years. What has changed is the scientific basis underpinning this advice. The rationale has shifted as more has become known of the factors which influence the development of chronic diseases.

In the 1970s and 1980s, fruit and vegetables were promoted alongside whole grain cereals as a source of dietary fibre and a 'gap-filler' to make up for the calories lost by cutting back on fat. In the United States in the 1980s, fruit and vegetables began to be promoted for their protective effects against cancer, but there was uncertainty about the precise reasons why high intakes of vegetables and fruits were associated with lower rates of cancer. By the 1990s, most dietary recommendations explicitly recommended vegetables and fruits to help protect against cancer, but remained cautious about the specific role of antioxidant nutrients. It was only in the mid-1990s that dietary recommendations began to acknowledge the role of vegetables and fruits, and the antioxidant nutrients they contain, in relation to the prevention of coronary heart disease.

This chapter summarises and traces the development of the recommendations on fruit and vegetables, concentrating on recommendations from international organisations and national agencies in the UK and the United States. Table 1 (on page 58) gives a summary of dietary recommendations and the reasons behind them from national and international reports from 1973 to 1994. Table 2 (on page 60) summarises the dietary guidelines with an assessment of the relationship between coronary heart disease and cancer with vegetables and fruits and antioxidants.

Population-wide recommendations on vegetables and fruit

Throughout the history of diet and nutrition education, 'vegetables and fruits' have been identified as a separate food group and seen as a source of vitamins or 'protective factors'. In 1921, when the discovery and understanding of the role of vitamins was in its infancy, the UK Ministry of Health report on *Diet in Relation to Normal Nutrition*[4] stated that it was necessary to supplement basic diets with vegetables to provide 'protective factors' to prevent deficiency diseases. During the Second World War, when Britain had a specific Ministry of Food, promotion of the production and consumption of domestic vegetables was based on their 'protective properties'.[5] Slogans such as these were used:

> *"Veg means vitamins, so keep your 'vits' about you."*
> *"You can look right if you feel right, and you can feel right if you eat right. An ounce of cabbage is worth an inch of lipstick."*

The role of 'protective factors' continued to be a cornerstone of dietary advice and formed a major component of the British Medical Association's report on diet and health in 1950.[6]

Vegetables and fruits to replace fatty foods

American Heart Association, 1973

Rising coronary heart disease death rates in the post-war period prompted an interest in diet and prevention. For many years the focus in dietary guidelines was primarily on reducing dietary fat intakes. The American Heart Association (AHA),[7] a professional organisation committed to the prevention of coronary heart disease in the United States, began producing dietary recommendations advising a reduction in fat and saturated fat in 1961. The AHA's Nutrition Committee regularly reviewed and updated its recommendations to take account of new scientific evidence, producing new public statements every three to five years. Statements in 1973, 1978 and 1982 additionally recommended that saturated fats should be replaced by polyunsaturated fats and complex carbohydrates, "as contained in cereals, beans, vegetables and some fruits" (see Table 1 on page 58). This reference to complex carbohydrates was based on early studies showing that substituting saturated fats in the diet with complex carbohydrates usually produced a fall in plasma and low density lipoprotein (LDL) cholesterol. The lower plasma triglycerides of populations which habitually consume diets rich in carbohydrates was also noted. The AHA recommendation emphasised complex carbohydrates because they imparted less risk of dental caries, provided more roughage and helped avoid hypoglycaemia.

In common with other dietary recommendations on coronary heart disease prevention at the time, the AHA's recommendations during the 1970s focused entirely on reducing fat intakes and plasma cholesterol levels. In 1982, the

AHA's review notes that dietary factors unrelated to plasma cholesterol and lipid levels may be linked with risk of coronary heart disease. It points to the results of the Seven Countries Study where, at similar serum cholesterol levels, Mediterranean men had a much lower risk of coronary heart disease compared with men from Finland and the United States. Scientists began to question whether factors in addition to or apart from fat were involved.

Royal College of Physicians of London, 1976
In Britain, one of the earliest recommendations on vegetables and fruits in the context of chronic disease prevention came from the Royal College of Physicians' (RCP) report on *Prevention of Coronary Heart Disease* in 1976.[8] This followed the UK government's advisory committee, the Committee on Medical Aspects of Food Policy's (COMA) report on *Diet and Coronary Heart Disease*[9] in 1974 which recommended reducing intakes of fat and saturated fatty acids. The RCP report went several stages further than COMA. Quantified targets for fat reduction were developed and the practical implications of the recommendations for individual diets were examined. The advice was to eat more vegetables and fruits in order to achieve the recommended reductions in fat intake. This strategy of recommending vegetables and fruits to make up for the decrease in calorie intake resulting from reducing fat intakes continued to underpin most of the subsequent dietary recommendations published in Britain until 1993.

National Advisory Committee on Nutrition Education, 1983
In the mid-1970s, the UK Secretary of State for Health and Social Services began an initiative to improve nutrition education. This led to the establishment of a multi-sectoral National Advisory Committee on Nutrition Education (NACNE). NACNE's report, *Proposals for Nutritional Guidelines for Health Education in Britain,*[10] published in 1983, drew together recommendations from previous expert committees and made practical proposals for implementing these recommendations. This included a recommendation to increase consumption of bread, potatoes, vegetables and fruits by 25%-30% each, in order to maintain energy levels and compensate for reducing fat and refined sugar intakes. NACNE estimated that a decrease of around 155kcal per person per day from fat and sugar was needed, and proposed that this could be replaced by an extra 70-100kcal from bread, 30-40kcal from potatoes and 30-40kcal from vegetables and fruits. NACNE added that these changes would also have the desirable effect of increasing dietary fibre. (A separate recommendation to increase fibre intakes by around 25% was based on a consideration of metabolic studies on the effects of dietary fibre on faecal weight and epidemiological evidence on intakes of dietary fibre and incidence of irritable bowel syndrome, constipation, diverticulosis and colon cancer.)

Diet and Cardiovascular Disease, COMA, 1984
A year later, the report of the Committee on Medical Aspects of Food Policy (COMA) on *Diet and Cardiovascular Disease*[11] similarly advised the public to compensate for reducing fat intakes by eating more fibre-rich carbohydrates such as bread, cereal, vegetables and fruits. This was largely based on the principle of caloric compensation with low fat foods, although the report acknowledged that increasing fibre intakes may be beneficial for other, non-cardiovascular, conditions. COMA reviewed epidemiological evidence from

studies carried out in the UK, Puerto Rico, Hawaii and the Netherlands which suggested that high intakes of dietary fibre or complex carbohydrates are associated with a reduced incidence of coronary heart disease. However, it concluded that the protective effect of fibre against coronary heart disease had not been adequately tested.

Vegetables and fruits as sources of vitamins A and C

Diet, Nutrition and Cancer, National Academy of Sciences, United States, 1982
The National Cancer Institute (NCI), a US government agency, has played a pivotal role in drawing attention to the role of vegetables and fruits in chronic disease prevention. The NCI established a specific programme on diet and cancer and in 1980 commissioned a comprehensive review of the scientific evidence, from the National Academy of Sciences (NAS). The report of the NAS's Committee, *Diet, Nutrition and Cancer,* published in 1982, marked a turning point and influenced many subsequent dietary recommendations both in the United States and worldwide.[12] The NAS Committee was the first to recommend increased consumption of vegetables and fruits based on their nutritive and non-nutritive constituents, rather than displacing fatty foods. At the time, there was no reference to 'antioxidant nutrients' and there was uncertainty over precisely which components of vegetables and fruits were responsible for the protective effect.

The Committee found persuasive evidence for advocating consumption of foods rich in vitamin A (and its precursors) and vitamin C. This was based on laboratory evidence of the ability of these vitamins to suppress induced tumours, and epidemiological evidence of an inverse relationship between risk of cancer and consumption of foods rich in these vitamins. However, the epidemiological evidence also suggested that other bioactive compounds in certain vegetables were associated with the reduced risk of cancer and some of these compounds had been shown to inhibit carcinogenesis in laboratory animals. On this basis, rather than recommending specific nutrients, the Committee favoured emphasising vegetables and fruits, especially carotene-rich and cruciferous vegetables (vegetables in the cabbage family such as sprouts, spring greens and cabbage), and fruits, especially citrus fruits high in vitamin C. The Committee drew no firm conclusions on vitamin E. It noted that, because vitamin E is present in many commonly consumed foods, it is difficult to identify populations with substantially different intakes, and consequently there were few epidemiological reports on vitamin E intake and risk of cancer. The Committee found evidence for the protective effect of fibre against colorectal cancer inconclusive. They pointed to the conflicting results of case control and cohort studies and the difficulty of equating laboratory studies which investigate the effects of specific components of fibre, with epidemiological studies based on estimates of total fibre intake which include a heterogeneous mixture of compounds.

Mediterranean intakes of vegetables and fruits

World Health Organization, 1982
In 1982, the World Health Organization's report on *Prevention of Coronary Heart Disease*[13] recommended increasing consumption of vegetables and fruits but from a very different perspective. WHO recommended that dietary guidelines

should emphasise foods of plant origin, vegetables, fruit, whole grains and legumes, to increase complex carbohydrate intake and to emulate the diets characteristic of populations with low rates of coronary heart disease. This approach is rooted in a consideration of the epidemiology of coronary heart disease rather than the identification of any particular protective properties contained in vegetables and fruits.

Rationale for the recommendations until the early 1980s

By 1982, three main reasons were given for recommending increased fruit and vegetable consumption:

- to replace the calories lost by reducing fat (and sugar) intakes and to provide fibre to prevent constipation and diverticulosis (found in most reports concerned with prevention of coronary heart disease);

- to emulate diets of populations with low rates of coronary heart disease (found in WHO's report on prevention of coronary heart disease);

- to provide vitamins A and C and other non-nutritive substances which seem to be protective against cancer (found in the US National Academy of Science report on diet and cancer).

Uncertainty on antioxidants and cancer

Whereas the American Cancer Society (ACS) and NCI made strong recommendations on the role of vegetables and fruits in lowering the risk of cancer, other bodies were noticeably more reticent. A report of an international workshop on diet and cancer held by the European Cancer Prevention Organisation and International Union of Nutritional Sciences published in 1986[14] concluded that "the evidence relating diet to human cancer was not as strong or consistent as desirable". However, it was considered prudent to advocate greater consumption of vegetables and fruits which have a high content of carotene and vitamin C because this was "consonant with recommendations for the prevention of CHD".

The NCI[15] and ACS[16] successively reviewed the epidemiological evidence published after the 1982 NAS report and revised their recommendations accordingly. The NCI made amendments to its dietary guidelines in 1984, to reflect increased epidemiological evidence that a dietary pattern of high fibre foods is inversely related to colon cancer. A specific recommendation to eat foods that provide 25-35g* of fibre was introduced. The ACS was more guarded, stating that although agreement on fibre's role in cancer protection was not universal, foods high in fibre could be recommended as a "wholesome substitute" for fatty foods. In 1988, the NCI's previous recommendation on fruit, vegetables and whole grain foods was altered to exclude whole grain foods and stress the importance of including vegetables and fruits in the daily diet. This reflected a strengthening of evidence for the protective effect of diets high in vegetables and fruits independent of their fibre content. The 1988 revision acknowledged evidence that carotenoids, rather than total vitamin A, were associated with a lower risk of lung cancer. Many previous

---

*   These figures are derived from the Southgate measure of fibre. They are substantially in excess of new numbers developed from Englyst's analyses.

epidemiological studies did not distinguish between the effects of dietary carotenoids and pre-formed vitamin A. Also in 1988, the NCI funded a pilot programme in California promoting fruit and vegetables, based on eating *5 A Day – for Better Health*. (For more details see *At Least Five a Day: Strategies to Increase Fruit and Vegetable Consumption*.[17])

Surgeon General's Report, United States, 1988
The US *Surgeon General's Report on Nutrition and Health* (1988)[18] was more cautious than the NCI in its interpretation of the evidence on diet and cancer. It found the evidence on increased fibre intakes and risk of colon cancer inconclusive, pointing out that other factors in high fibre diets may be responsible. It noted evidence which suggested that frequent consumption of vegetables and fruit, particularly dark green, deep yellow and cruciferous vegetables may lower the risk of some cancers, but that the specific components which might be responsible had not been established. However the Surgeon General's report was concerned with nutrition and general health, not just cancer and, on balance, concluded that "current evidence suggests it would be prudent to increase consumption of wholegrain foods and cereals, vegetables (including beans and peas) and fruits". This was based on a consideration of the role of high fibre diets in preventing constipation and diverticular disease. On coronary heart disease, the report describes the difficulty of interpreting evidence of an association between diets high in complex carbohydrates and fruits and vegetables as these also tended to be lower in fat. This is further confused by evidence that certain types of dietary fibre in oats and some fruits were associated with lower blood cholesterol levels.

Introduction of quantified advice
Quantified advice on fruit and vegetable consumption was first introduced in the late 1980s.

Diet and Health, National Research Council, United States, 1989
In 1989, the Committee on Diet and Health of the US National Research Council (NRC) published a comprehensive report, *Diet and Health: Implications for Reducing Chronic Disease Risk*.[19] This made recommendations to "eat five or more servings of a combination of vegetables and fruit, especially green and yellow vegetables and citrus fruits, and increase consumption of starches and other complex carbohydrates by eating six or more daily servings of bread, cereals and legumes". This recommendation was based on a broad consideration of the role of plant-based foods in the US diet, including their potential as a low fat substitute for fatty foods. The recommended number of servings was set pragmatically, based on experience of planning nutritionally balanced diets that would meet all of the committee's dietary recommendations.

The NRC found persuasive the epidemiological evidence that diets high in plant-based foods were associated with low rates of coronary heart disease and cancer, but did not draw many firm conclusions about the agents responsible. It concluded that the usually low saturated fat and cholesterol content of diets rich in plant-derived foods largely explained lower rates of coronary heart disease, although some other constituents such as soluble fibre might also be involved. It noted that there was good evidence of a link between low consumption levels of beta-carotene and high rates of lung cancer, and also between low levels of vitamin C and an increased incidence of stomach cancer. Thus, epidemiological evidence supported greater consumption of green and yellow vegetables and citrus fruits.

In 1990, the ACS[20] toned down their 1984 recommendation which specifically referred to cruciferous vegetables and vitamins A and C. They replaced this with a general statement about vegetables and fruits. Eighteen months later, the ACS[21] made further minor revisions to their recommendations, stressing that the daily diet should include 'both' fruit and vegetables, and removed all mention of vitamins A or C in the supporting text.

World Health Organization, 1990
In the 1990 WHO report *Diet, Nutrition and the Prevention of Chronic Diseases*,[22] a diet relatively rich in vegetables and fruits was recommended. This was based on emulating intakes of fruit and vegetables in countries with low rates of coronary heart disease and some cancers. In reviewing the evidence on the links between diet and coronary heart disease, the WHO Committee commented that the dietary factors which affect serum cholesterol tend to cluster together in many diets. This made it difficult to ascertain if the lower rates of coronary heart disease found in population subgroups consuming a vegetarian diet were caused by the low fat content of the diet, or by the high fibre content, or if they were due to some other factor. The report found consistency in the evidence that vegetables and fruit, especially green and yellow vegetables and citrus fruits, play some protective role in preventing the development of cancers. Although the mechanisms underlying these effects were not fully understood, the Committee noted the lack of conclusive evidence for a beneficial effect due to the high fibre content of plant-derived foods. The Committee stated that other factors, such as vitamins E, C and beta-carotene, may be involved.

The WHO Committee adopted a new approach by developing a series of 'population nutrient goals' – mean population intakes which were judged to be consistent with good health and the prevention of chronic diseases. These were intended for use in all parts of the world, and were expressed as upper and lower limits, recognising that there was a range of healthy mean intakes. The Committee recommended a lower limit of 400g of vegetables and fruits (excluding tubers), including at least 30g of pulses, nuts and seeds. No upper limit was set. This 400g goal was set 'judgementally' based on apparently healthy fruit and vegetable intakes of populations living in countries with low rates of coronary heart disease on the north coast of the Mediterranean. By developing a 'population nutrient goal' which referred to foods, rather than nutrients, the Committee broke new ground.

Healthy People 2000, United States, 1991
In 1991, the US government developed national health promotion and disease prevention objectives[23] drawing on the recommendations of previous expert committees. These included an objective to increase consumption of complex carbohydrate and fibre-containing foods to five or more daily servings of vegetables and fruit, and six or more daily servings of grain products. This was based on the value of plant-derived foods as a source of complex carbohydrate, dietary fibre and vitamins and minerals, and their potential as a

substitute for foods high in fat. The recommendation was framed to increase consumption of fibre-rich foods, referring to evidence for a protective effect of fibre-rich foods against colon cancer. There was little mention of any possible role for antioxidant nutrients in lowering the risk of cancer. On coronary heart disease, the report repeated the reservations of the Surgeon General's report in 1988. It pointed to the difficulty of interpreting epidemiological studies of diets rich in plant-based foods and coronary heart disease because such diets were also low in fat. Interestingly, the quantitative objective on fruit and vegetables is repeated in a separate section of the report which deals with cancer, but not in the section on coronary heart disease.

In 1991, the NCI's pilot *5 A Day – for Better Health* campaign became a national collaboration between NCI and the fruit and vegetable industry.[17] In 1992, the United States' national food guide, the 'food pyramid' which offered practical advice on implementing the dietary guidelines for Americans, advised consumption of between five and nine servings of fruit and vegetables a day depending on size and activity levels.[24]

For more information on the formulation of quantified advice for vegetable and fruit consumption, see Chapter 6.

Antioxidant nutrients and cardiovascular diseases

The Scottish Diet, 1993
The first national report in the UK to link the role of antioxidant nutrients in vegetables and fruits to both cancer and coronary heart disease was *The Scottish Diet* report,[25] the report of a working group set up under the Scottish Office national strategy for health, *Scotland's Health: A Challenge to Us All*. The report described the hypothesis that antioxidant nutrients help combat LDL oxidation. It outlined the epidemiological evidence suggesting that differences in death rates from coronary heart disease across western Europe may relate to the ratio of LDL cholesterol and the plasma content of the dietary antioxidants, beta-carotene, vitamin C and alpha-tocopherol (vitamin E). On cancer, the working group referred to a recent collation of over 200 case control studies which strongly suggested that a high vegetable and fruit intake was associated with a two- to four-fold reduction in the risk of many cancers. A large number of components in vegetables and fruit may be responsible for this effect, including compounds which act as antioxidants. The group concluded that the epidemiological evidence was now sufficiently clear to warrant advice to the Scottish public to alter their diet by doubling their fruit and vegetable intake.

The report proposed that Scotland's population should eat, every day, an average of over 400g of vegetables and fruit. It noted that this is similar to the 400g figure chosen by WHO, and although more recent analysis of the diets of southern Italians suggests that intakes are in practice higher, it saw no reason to depart from this figure.

Nutritional Aspects of Cardiovascular Disease, COMA, 1994
The COMA report on *Nutritional Aspects of Cardiovascular Disease*, published at the end of 1994, considered the role of antioxidants and cardiovascular disease in detail.[26] It concluded that evidence for the protective effect of the antioxidant vitamins E and C against susceptibility to atherosclerosis was "persuasive, but not yet conclusive" and noted that other substances in plant-based foods might be important.

The COMA report voiced concerns over the lack of evidence for the safety and efficacy of high-dose antioxidant supplements, but acknowledged that some studies suggest that to achieve beneficial effects, intakes of antioxidants greater than those which can be readily achieved by dietary means may be necessary. The report recommended that further research into antioxidant nutrients was needed and did not give a specific dietary goal for antioxidant nutrients. However, the section of the report dealing with the implications of the Committee's recommendations for foods includes a recommendation to increase fruit and vegetable consumption by 50%. This is both to increase dietary intakes of antioxidant nutrients and to replace the energy deficit resulting from reducing fat consumption. Substituting saturated animal fats with unsaturated vegetable oils was also recommended, which would have the effect of increasing intakes of vitamin E.

Summary of UK recommendations on vegetables and fruit

In reviewing past dietary recommendations on vegetables and fruits it is evident that, until recently, increasing consumption of antioxidant nutrients has been a minor consideration. The evidence on the role of antioxidant nutrients in protection against coronary heart disease as well as cancer, strengthens the basis for health recommendations to increase fruit and vegetable consumption. The main reasons for increasing fruit and vegetable consumption in the UK, according to national recommendations are:

- *Vegetables and fruits may be protective against chronic diseases such as cardiovascular diseases and many cancers.*
  This is partly attributed to the antioxidant vitamins A (carotenoids), C, and E, but other bioactive constituents of fruit and vegetables are probably also involved.

- *To increase intakes of dietary fibre.*
  Current average fibre intakes are around 12.5g compared with a desirable average intake of 18g.[27]* High fibre intakes help in the management of constipation and diverticulosis and are associated with lower risk of colon cancer.

- *Vegetables and fruits can improve the nutritional quality of the diet.*
  They provide vitamins and minerals and fibre and, by displacing other less nutritious fatty and sugary foods from the diet, they can reduce the proportion of energy derived from fat and sugar.

- *Vegetables and fruits are bulky and have a relatively low energy density (number of calories per 100g of food).*
  Eating low energy dense foods can assist in weight reduction. In England, in 1994, more than half (56%) of men, and 45% of women were overweight (body mass index over 25). Thirteen per cent of men and 16% of women are obese (body mass index over 30).

---

* These figures are derived using the nomenclature and analytical methods developed by Englyst.

Table 1   Summary chronology: key recommendations on fruits and vegetables for the UK and United States

Date	Organisation/Report	Recommendation	Reason
1973 1975 1982	American Heart Association	Eat more complex carbohydrates as contained in vegetables, beans, cereals and some fruits.	Compensate for calorie deficit of reducing fat intake to a maximum of 30% energy.
1974	Committee on Medical Aspects of Food Policy (COMA) *Diet and Coronary Heart Disease*[9]		No mention of fruit and vegetables. Concern over association between rising intakes of simple sugars and coronary heart disease rates.
1976	Royal College of Physicians/ British Cardiac Society *Prevention of Coronary Heart Disease*[8]	Eat more fruit and vegetables of all kinds.	As a means to achieve fat reduction target.
1982	National Academy of Sciences, United States *Diet, Nutrition and Cancer*[12]	Emphasise the importance of including fruit, vegetables and whole grain cereals in the daily diet.	Epidemiological evidence that increased consumption of certain vegetables, especially carotene-rich and cruciferous vegetables, and fruits, especially citrus fruits rich in vitamin C, is associated with a lower incidence of cancer at several sites.
1982	World Health Organization *Prevention of Coronary Heart Disease*[13]	Emphasise appropriately combined foods of plant origin: beans, cereals, grains, vegetables (cooked and raw) and fruit.	To increase carbohydrate intake and to emulate diets characteristic of populations with low rates of coronary heart disease.
1983	National Advisory Committee on Nutrition Education (NACNE) *Proposals for Nutritional Guidelines for Health Education in Britain*[10]	Increase intake of bread, potatoes, fruit and vegetables by 25%-30% each.	Compensate for calorie deficit of reducing fat and sugar intakes. Estimate total deficit of 155kcal lost. Extra fruit and vegetables to make up 30-40kcal. Increase fibre levels to prevent constipation, diverticulosis etc.
1984	American Cancer Society *Nutrition and Cancer: Causes and Prevention*[16]	Eat more high fibre foods such as whole grain cereals, fruits and vegetables. Include foods rich in vitamins A and C, and cruciferous vegetables in the daily diet.	Fibre-rich foods are a good substitute for fatty foods, and fibre may have a role in cancer prevention. Diets high in vitamins A, C and cruciferous vegetables associated with a lower risk of cancer.
1984	National Cancer Institute, United States	Include fresh fruits, vegetables and whole grain cereals in the daily diet.	Increase intakes of fibre as well as carotenoids, vitamin C and other non-nutritive substances which reduce risk of cancer.
1984	Committee on Medical Aspects of Food Policy *Diet and Cardiovascular Disease*[11]	Increase intake of fibre-rich carbohydrates, eg bread, cereals, fruit and vegetables.	Compensate for a reduced fat intake.
1986	European Cancer Prevention Organisation and International Union of Nutritional Sciences *Workshop on Diet and Human Carcinogenesis*[14]	Eat a varied diet containing different types of vegetables and fruit, especially leafy green and root vegetables and citrus fruits.	Evidence on cancer and fruit and vegetables not strong, but prudent advice consonant with recommendations to protect against coronary heart disease.
1988	National Cancer Institute, United States *Dietary Guidelines*[15]	Include a variety of vegetables and fruits in the daily diet.	As 1984, but recognising the role of fruit and vegetables independent of fibre content.

Date	Organisation/Report	Recommendation	Reason
1988	Surgeon General's Report, United States[18]	Increase consumption of whole grain foods, and cereal products, vegetables (including dried beans and peas) and fruits.	Raise fibre and complex carbohydrate intake to help management of constipation and diverticulosis. Fruit and vegetables may lower risk of cancer.
1989	National Research Council, United States *Diet and Health: Implications for Reducing Chronic Disease Risk*[19]	Every day eat five or more servings of a combination of vegetables and fruits, especially green and yellow vegetables and citrus fruits. Increase intake of starches and other complex carbohydrates by eating six or more daily servings of a combination of breads, cereals or legumes.	Diets high in fruit and vegetables are associated with low risk of coronary heart disease. As a low fat substitute for fatty foods. Soluble fibre may lower blood cholesterol levels. Diets high in fruit and vegetables, especially green and yellow vegetables and citrus fruits, are associated with low susceptibility to certain cancers.
1990	American Cancer Society *Guidelines on Diet, Nutrition and Cancer*[21]	Include a variety of vegetables and fruits in the daily diet. Eat more high fibre foods such as whole grain cereals, vegetables and fruits.	As 1984, except emphasis is on fruit and vegetables in general rather than vitamins A and C and cruciferous vegetables.
1990	United States Department of Agriculture/Department of Health and Human Services *Dietary Guidelines for Americans*	Eat at least three servings of vegetables and two servings of fruit daily.	
1990	World Health Organization *Diet, Nutrition and the Prevention of Chronic Diseases*[22]	Population Nutrient Goal lower limit of 400g of fruit and vegetables a day, including 30g of pulses, nuts and seeds. To avoid significant risk of inadequacy, population should have a higher mean intake, so that most of the population consume a minimum of 400g a day.	Contribute to balancing the diet because they are high in fibre, vitamins and minerals and low in energy and fat. Evidence of a protective role against cancer, independent of their fibre content. Improve availability of iron and reduce vitamin A deficiency. Emulate diets of populations with low rates of coronary heart disease.
1991	Department of Health and Human Services, United States *Healthy People 2000*[23]	Increase complex carbohydrate and fibre-containing foods in the diets of adults, to five or more daily servings for vegetables (including legumes) and fruits, and to six or more servings for grain products.	Good source of complex carbohydrate, fibre, vitamins and minerals. Substitute for foods high in fat. Associated with lower risk of cancer.
1991	Ministry of Agriculture, Fisheries and Food *Eight Guidelines for a Healthy Diet*	Try to eat some vegetables or fruit at every meal.	Provide valuable vitamins, minerals and fibre with little fat.
1992	United States Department of Agriculture *Food Pyramid Food Guide*[24]	3-5 servings of vegetables a day 2-4 servings of fruit a day	Based on USDA/DHHS *Dietary Guidelines for Americans*.
1993	Scottish Office *The Scottish Diet*[25]	Double intake of fresh and frozen vegetables, and fresh fruit. Achieve daily average population intake of over 400g.	Evidence of protective effect of fruit and vegetables against coronary heart disease and cancer, possible role against stroke, hypertension, overweight. Based partly on antioxidant mechanism.
1994	Committee on Medical Aspects of Food Policy (COMA) *Nutritional Aspects of Cardiovascular Disease*[26]	Increase average population intakes of fruit and vegetables by 50%.	Evidence of the protective effect of diets high in fruit and vegetables, possibly due to their antioxidant content. Make up energy deficit resulting from reducing fat consumption.

Table 2 *Summary of conclusions of expert reports on the relationship between fruit and vegetables and the antioxidant vitamins with coronary heart disease and cancer*

This table uses standard terms to summarise the conclusions of the different expert reports on the strength of the evidence for an association between diet and disease. These are not the terms that were necessarily used in each of the reports, but are based on the authors' assessment of the expert committees' conclusions based on the discussion in the text of the report. Where items were not mentioned in a report, the entry has been left blank.

Yes = Convincing evidence of a direct relationship

Probably = Evidence strong enough to conclude that a direct relationship is likely

Possibly = Consistent evidence of a relationship exists, but is not strong

Uncertain = Evidence unclear

	CORONARY HEART DISEASE				
	Fruit & vegetables	Beta-carotene	Vitamin C	Vitamin E	Dietary fibre
1988 Surgeon General's Report, United States[18]	Possibly – maybe fat displacement or soluble fibre	Insufficient evidence	Insufficient evidence	Possibly soluble fibre – clinical studies	
1989 National Research Council, United States *Diet and Health: Implications for Reducing Chronic Disease Risk*[19]	Yes – probably fat displacement				Possibly soluble fibre – clinical studies and laboratory studies
1990 World Health Organization *Diet, Nutrition and the Prevention of Chronic Diseases*[22]	Possibly				Uncertain
1991 US Dept of Agriculture/ Dept of Health and Human Services *Healthy People 2000*[23]	Yes – maybe fat displacement or soluble fibre				Probably soluble fibre – clinical studies
1993 Scottish Office *The Scottish Diet*[25]	Yes	Yes	Yes	Yes	
1994 Committee on Medical Aspects of Food Policy (COMA) *Nutritional Aspects of Cardiovascular Disease*[26]	Yes – epidemiological evidence and fat displacement	No	Probably	Probably	Yes – soluble fibre

Epidemiol. = Epidemiological

	CANCER						
	Fruit & vegetables	Retinol	Beta-carotene	Vitamin C	Vitamin E	Non-nutritive compounds	Dietary fibre
1982 National Academy of Sciences, United States *Diet, Nutrition and Cancer*[12]	Yes – epidemiol. evidence	Yes – epidemiol. evidence & laboratory studies	Yes – epidemiol. evidence	Yes – laboratory. Probably – epidemiol. evidence	Insufficient evidence	Yes – epidemiol. evidence	No – epidemiol. evidence and laboratory studies
1984 American Cancer Society *Nutrition and Cancer: Causes and Prevention*[16]	Yes	Possibly – epidemiol. evidence. Yes – laboratory studies	Possibly – epidemiol. evidence	Probably – epidemiol. evidence	No	Yes – epidemiol. evidence and laboratory studies	Uncertain
1988 Surgeon General's Report, United States[18]	Possibly		Possibly	Possibly	Possibly	Probably – epidemiol. evidence	Possibly – colon cancer
1988 National Cancer Institute, US *Dietary Guidelines*[15]	Yes	Probably no	Probably – epidemiol. evidence	Possibly	Uncertain	Probably – epidemiol. evidence	Yes – colon cancer. Uncertain – other cancers
1989 National Research Council, United States *Diet and Health: Implications for Reducing Chronic Disease Risk*[19]	Yes – maybe fat displacement	No – epidemiol. evidence. Yes – laboratory studies	Yes – epidemiol. evidence lung cancer	Yes – stomach cancer – epidemiol. evidence and laboratory studies. Uncertain – other cancers	Insufficient evidence	Probably	
1990 American Cancer Society *Guidelines on Diet, Nutrition and Cancer*[21]	Yes – epidemiol. evidence	Uncertain	Uncertain	Probably – epidemiol. evidence	Insufficient evidence	Possibly	Uncertain
1990 World Health Organization *Diet, Nutrition and the Prevention of Chronic Diseases*[22]	Yes – epidemiol. evidence		Possibly	Possibly	Possibly	Possibly	Uncertain
1991 US Dept of Agriculture/Dept of Health and Human Services *Healthy People 2000*[23]	Yes – epidemiol. evidence		Possibly			Possibly	Yes – colon cancer. Uncertain – other cancers
1993 Scottish Office *The Scottish Diet*[25]	Yes		Possibly	Possibly	Possibly	Yes	Yes

References

1   Diplock AT. 1994. Antioxidants and disease prevention. *Molecular Aspects of Disease*; 15: 4. Pergamon Press.

2   Steinmetz KA, Potter JD. 1993. Vegetables, fruit and cancer. II. Mechanisms. *Cancer Causes and Control*; 2: 427-442.

3   Steinmetz KA, Potter JD. 1993. Vegetables, fruit and cancer. I. Epidemiology. *Cancer Causes and Control*; 2: 325-357.

4   Hamill JM. 1921. *Diet in Relation to Normal Nutrition. Report on Public Health and Medical Subjects (9).* London: HMSO.

5   Davies J. 1993. *The Wartime Kitchen and Garden: The Home Front 1939-1945.* London: BBC Books.

6   British Medical Association. 1950. *Report of the Committee on Nutrition.* London: British Medical Association.

7   American Heart Association. 1982. Rationale of the Diet-Heart Statement of the American Heart Association. Report of the AHA Nutrition Committee. *Arteriosclerosis*; 4: 177-191.

8   Royal College of Physicians of London/British Cardiac Society. 1976. Prevention of Coronary Heart Disease. *Journal of the Royal College of Physicians*; 10 (3): 1-63.

9   Department of Health and Social Security. 1974. *Diet and Coronary Heart Disease. Report of the Advisory Panel of the Committee on Medical Aspects of Food Policy (Nutrition). Report on Health and Social Subjects 7.* London: HMSO.

10 National Advisory Committee on Nutrition Education (NACNE). 1983. *Proposals for Nutritional Guidelines for Health Education in Britain.* London: Health Education Council.

11 Department of Health. 1984. *Diet and Cardiovascular Disease. Committee on Medical Aspects of Food Policy: Report of the Panel on Diet in Relation to Cardiovascular Disease. Report on Health and Social Subjects 28.* London: HMSO.

12 National Academy of Sciences Committee on Diet, Nutrition and Cancer. Assembly of Life Sciences, National Research Council. 1982. *Diet, Nutrition and Cancer.* Washington DC: National Academy Press.

13 World Health Organization. 1982. *Prevention of Coronary Heart Disease. Report of a WHO Expert Committee. WHO Technical Report Series 1982 (678).* Geneva: World Health Organization.

14 Proceedings of a Joint ECP - IUNS workshop on Diet and Human Carcinogenesis (Arrhus, Denmark, June 1985). 1986. *Nutrition and Cancer*; 8 (1): 17-21.

15 Butrum RR, Clifford CC, Lanza E. 1988. NCI dietary guidelines: rationale. *American Journal of Clinical Nutrition*; 48: 888-895.

16 American Cancer Society. Special report. Nutrition and cancer: causes and prevention. CA-A. *Cancer Journal for Clinicians*, 1984; 34 (2): 121-126.

17 National Heart Forum. 1997. *At Least Five a Day: Strategies to Increase Fruit and Vegetable Consumption.* London: The Stationery Office.

18 US Dept. of Health and Human Services. 1988. *The Surgeon General's Report on Nutrition and Health. DHHS (PHS) Publication No. 88-50210.* Washington DC: US Government Printing Office.

19 Committee on Diet and Health, Food and Nutrition Board, National Research Council (US). 1989. *Diet and Health: Implications for Reducing Chronic Disease Risk.* Washington DC: National Academy Press.

20 Nixon DW. 1990. Nutrition and cancer: American Cancer Society guidelines, programs and initiatives. CA-A *Cancer Journal for Clinicians*; 40 (2): 71-75.

21 American Cancer Society. 1991. Guidelines on Diet, Nutrition and Cancer. CA-A *Cancer Journal for Clinicians*; 41 (6): 334-338.

22 World Health Organization. 1990. *Diet, Nutrition and the Prevention of Chronic Diseases. WHO Technical Report Series 1990 (797).* Geneva: World Health Organization.

23 United States Department of Health and Human Services. 1991. *Healthy People 2000: National Health Promotion and Disease Prevention Objectives. DHHS (PHS) Publication No. DHS-91-50213.* Washington DC: US Government Printing Office.

24 *The Food Pyramid Food Guide. Beyond the Basic 4.* United States Department of Agriculture.

25 The Scottish Office. 1993. *The Scottish Diet. Report of a Working Party to the Chief Medical Officer for Scotland.* Edinburgh: The Scottish Office Home and Health Department/HMSO Scotland.

26 Department of Health. 1994. *Nutritional Aspects of Cardiovascular Disease. Report of the Cardiovascular Review Group, Committee on Medical Aspects of Food Policy. Report on Health and Social Subjects 46.* London: HMSO.

27 Department of Health. 1991. *Dietary Reference Values for Food, Energy and Nutrients for the United Kingdom. Report of the Panel on Dietary Reference Values of the Committee on Medical Aspects of Food Policy.* London: HMSO.

Chapter 6

At least five a day? Devising quantified dietary advice on vegetables and fruit

Carol Williams

Nutrition Consultant

Professor Michael Marmot

Department of Epidemiology and Public Health, University College London

Introduction

In recent years, nutrition education for the public has begun to include quantified advice on fruit and vegetable intakes, with recommendations of 'five a day' or 'at least five a day'. This chapter examines the formulation of quantified advice on vegetables and fruit, and touches on the antioxidant nutrient, fruit and vegetable consumption patterns in the UK.

The principles underlying quantified advice on fruit and vegetables

Dietary recommendations can take two forms: recommendations for changes at the population level intended for policy makers, and recommendations for the general public on the changes required at the individual level to achieve the population goal. Early recommendations on vegetables and fruits, both at population and individual levels, simply advocated greater consumption. Policy makers were advised to seek an increase in overall consumption and the general public was advised to 'eat more'.

Where dietary recommendations on vegetables and fruits have been quantified and healthy levels of fruit and vegetable intakes suggested, these have been derived according to three distinct principles:

1   A practical consideration of the amounts needed for a 'balanced diet' which meets nutrient recommendations for fat, fibre, protein, vitamins and minerals. For example, the National Research Council[1] and *Healthy People 2000*,[2] both in the United States (see Chapter 5).

2   Using the epidemiological evidence on fruit and vegetable intakes in healthy populations with low rates of chronic diseases. For example, the dietary goal of the World Health Organization (WHO) of 400g of vegetables and fruits a day[3] or the 'at least 400g a day' recommendation of *The Scottish Diet* report.[4]

3   Judgement of what would represent a feasible, but significant change in the right direction. For example, the Committee on Medical Aspects of Food Policy (COMA) recommendation of a 50% increase in fruit and vegetables intake.[5]

Since the late 1980s, national agencies in the United States, and more recently in parts of the UK,[6] have recommended a target of 'at least five servings of vegetables and fruits a day'. This target is based on the amount of fruits and vegetables needed for a balanced diet, and is considered to be consistent with the epidemiological evidence of desirable intakes.[7] However, epidemiological studies of diet and disease tend to look at the weights of fruit and vegetables consumed. There appears to be no published review of healthy intakes measured by *frequency* of fruit and vegetable consumption. The WHO's 400g dietary goal would imply five servings of around 80g a day, which concurs well with average serving sizes of a wide range of fruits and vegetables in the UK diet*.[8] This rough translation of WHO's population goal has been used as the basis of 'five or more' or 'at least five' advice to the general public in the UK.[9]

In 1994, COMA conducted a review of diet and cardiovascular disease. COMA was committed to devising numerical targets because of their value as an objective measure for assessing progress, even if they had to be set using a pragmatic judgement. COMA considered that it was premature to recommend increased intakes of specific antioxidant nutrients, but recommended a 50% increase in fruit and vegetable intakes. This was based on their assessment of a feasible dietary change for the UK, rather than an intake which will lead to the lowest attainable rate of coronary heart disease. Since consumption of fruit and vegetables is estimated to be approximately 250g per day, achieving the COMA target would involve raising mean intakes to 375g of fruit and vegetables per person per day. To meet the recommendations of 400g or five portions of vegetables and fruits per day, an average increase in vegetable and fruit intakes of 60% is needed. For many people, a doubling (100% increase), or more, is required.

If the evidence for the protective effect of antioxidant nutrients against chronic diseases were strong enough, another approach to devising dietary recommendations on vegetables and fruit would be to base them on the intakes of antioxidant nutrients required to achieve a protective effect. This follows the standard approach to devising recommendations about foods and diets designed to provide sufficient amounts of vitamins or minerals to meet recommended daily amounts. These 'protective quantities' could be set using the levels of antioxidant nutrients found in healthy people who, according to the large observational and other epidemiological studies, are in the lowest risk quintile for coronary heart disease and cancer. Such an approach would

---

*   For example, a medium apple weighs 100g, a small banana 80g, a medium portion of broccoli 85g, a medium portion of carrots 60g, and a medium portion of peas 70g.

represent a paradigm shift in the setting of Dietary Reference Values (DRVs*) – from amounts of nutrients needed to prevent nutritional deficiencies, to amounts needed to promote optimal health. However, while this constitutes an interesting theoretical approach, there is insufficient evidence to use this method to make population-wide recommendations on antioxidant nutrients.

A nutrition education method of presenting dietary advice to the general public is by the use of 'food selection guides'. These provide a pictorial representation of a healthy, balanced diet (meeting all dietary recommendations, including recommended daily amounts for vitamins and minerals) broken down into different food groups. The *Food Pyramid Food Guide*,[10] published in the United States in 1992, recommends three to five servings from the vegetable group and two to four servings from the fruit group, depending on age, sex, size and activity. *The Balance of Good Health*,[11] published in the UK in 1994, does not provide written quantified advice on fruit and vegetable consumption. However, the proportions of the plate model occupied by the various food groups are intended to illustrate the proportion of the diet which should be derived from each food group. Fruit and vegetables occupy 33% of the plate model.

It is worth noting that WHO's 400g per day dietary goal expressly excludes potatoes and other starchy tubers eaten as a main starchy staple. Most recent dietary recommendations on vegetables and fruits in Britain, including *The Scottish Diet* report,[4] also exclude potatoes. In contrast, most of the recommendations on vegetables in the United States include baked or boiled potatoes, but tend not to feature potato crisps or chips. Potatoes provide a much larger proportion of carbohydrate in the British diet compared with the US. Diets in the United States place a greater reliance on bread, rice, cereals and pasta.

Why fruit and vegetables and not antioxidants?

Further research is needed to clarify which particular components of vegetables and fruits are responsible for their observed protective effect. While much attention in the media and lay press has been paid to antioxidant nutrients (recommending 'ACE' vitamins for health, for example), it is well recognised that vegetables and fruits contain bioactive microconstituents which probably have a key role. These have yet to be precisely identified or measured. These other components may act together and have a multiplicative or synergistic effect – an effect which would not be obtained from antioxidant vitamin supplements.

Even where there is a body of evidence relating to a particular nutrient, the situation is complicated by the numerous different types or homologues of the nutrient. Analysis of the carotenoids shows that among the 500 different carotenoids, many have completely different metabolic pathways. The 40-60 carotenoids with pro-vitamin A activity are transferred to the liver for storage as vitamin A. The other carotenoids are likely to be distributed peripherally in the

---

*   For an explanation of Dietary Reference Values, see Glossary on page 70.

tissues where they may act as a local source of antioxidants. Paradoxically, large doses of beta-carotene (a pro-vitamin A carotenoid) could actually prove harmful if they inhibited the absorption of these peripherally distributed antioxidants.[12]

The situation with regard to vitamin E is also complex. Vitamin E consists of a mixture of different tocopherols. It is derived from a variety of dietary sources (see Appendix) and is present in whole grain foods, nuts, seeds and green vegetables. However, the single largest dietary source in the UK is sunflower oil and products such as margarine and mayonnaise made with sunflower oil.

An analysis of vitamin E intakes in Europe by Belizzi et al,[13] based on the UN Food and Agriculture Organization's food supply data, indicates that the mean supply of alpha-tocopherol in France is 20.4mg per person per day, compared with a figure of 12mg in Britain. Belizzi et al propose that differences in alpha-tocopherol intake may be a factor in explaining what has become known as the 'French paradox' - low rates of coronary heart disease despite moderately high intakes of fat and saturated fats. They suggest that in many southern European countries an appreciable supply of total fat and saturated fats seems to be compatible with a low rate of coronary heart disease provided the supply of alpha-tocopherol is also high. So the type of tocopherol, rather than total vitamin E intake, may be important. Most of the difference in alpha-tocopherol intakes between France and the UK is explained by a far higher intake of sunflower oil which, contrary to popular opinion, is the predominant oil consumed in France, rather than olive oil.

Any recommendation to increase alpha-tocopherol intakes in the UK through increasing the proportion of dietary fats from sunflower oil would need to take account of COMA's recommendations on fat. These state that there should be no further increase in average intakes of polyunsaturated fatty acids (PUFAs) or the proportion of the population consuming more than 10% of dietary energy from polyunsaturates. This recommendation is based on a concern that high intakes of PUFAs may promote oxidative damage.

Are antioxidant supplements protective?

The results of studies using antioxidant supplements have been mixed, and there is some concern that specifying optimal levels of antioxidant nutrients might encourage people to use dietary supplements to achieve beneficial effects, rather than eating more fruit and vegetables. (For more details, see Chapter 2.)

Although apparently non-toxic, the long-term effects of a lifetime consumption of antioxidant supplements, in healthy people, is unknown. In addition, it is possible that no single level of antioxidant will be optimal at all times in all people. For example, it is known that tobacco smoke contains numerous compounds with oxidant potential and smoking has been shown to lower the level of vitamin C and beta-carotene in plasma. An added complication is that the diets of smokers are characteristically low in antioxidant vitamins and levels of fruit and vegetable consumption. Smokers may therefore need to consume higher amounts of antioxidants to achieve the same level of protection as non-smokers (see Chapter 2).

Other considerations include the stage at which the antioxidant supplements are given. For example, in cancer it appears that the stage at which a particular supplement is introduced may be crucial. Certain supplements given at a time when a cancer is proliferating may enhance rather than inhibit the cancer's development. The development of coronary heart disease is also a complex process and similar considerations may apply regarding the timing of administration and the dose of antioxidant supplements with stage of progress of disease. There is therefore a need for further long-term research into the effects of antioxidant supplements, including randomised controlled trials.

In contrast to the situation for antioxidant supplements, the long-term consumption of a diet rich in vegetables and fruit is known to be associated with a lower risk of chronic disease.

Intakes of antioxidant nutrients and vegetables and fruits

Intakes of antioxidant nutrients in the UK

The main sources of vitamin C and beta-carotene in the UK diet are fruit, vegetables and fruit juice. They provide around 80% of the vitamin C and 70% of beta-carotene (see Figure 1).

Figure 1 *Food sources of vitamins C, E and beta-carotene*

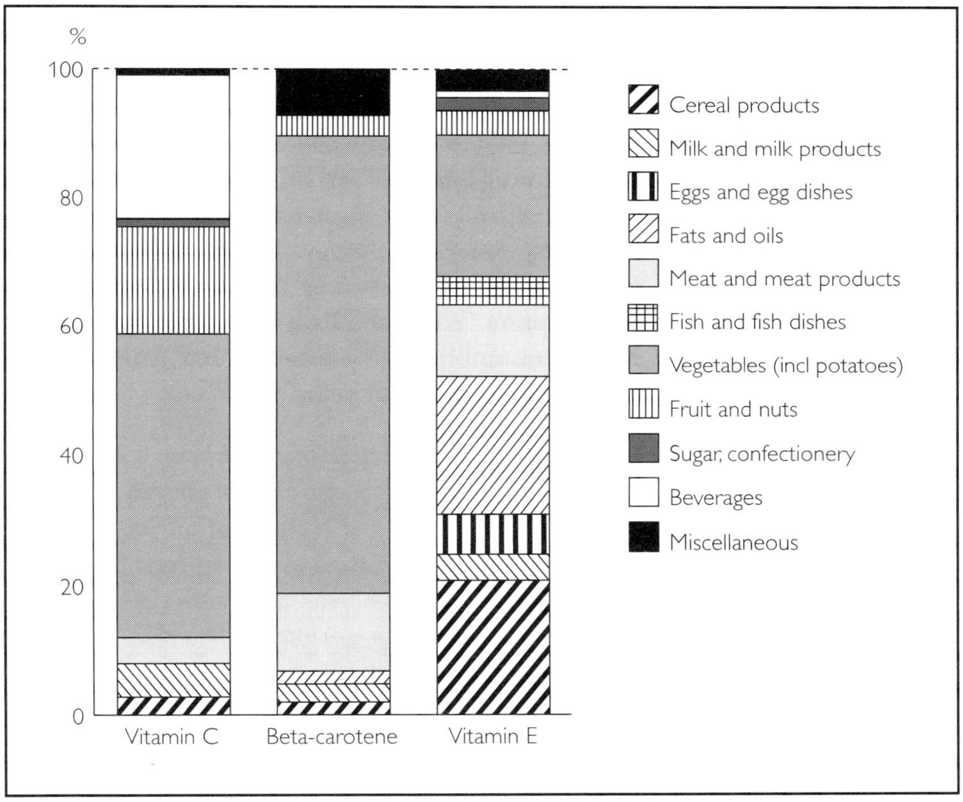

Source: See reference 14.

three-quarters of purchases by weight. The introduction of domestic freezers in the 1960s led to a steady increase in the proportion of frozen vegetables consumed, but in recent years the trend has been towards green and leafy salad vegetables.

Conclusion

When population-wide dietary recommendations are devised and revised, the state of scientific knowledge with regard to both coronary heart disease and cancer – the major causes of death and disability in the UK – needs to be taken into account. Only then is it possible to develop dietary strategies which offer the public maximum protection against chronic diseases. Dietary advice and nutrition information based on these recommendations need to be coherent and consistent if they are to be credible. This means that the relationship between new recommendations and previous dietary advice needs to be acknowledged, and any inconsistencies or changes need to be explained and justified.

There is strong scientific evidence to support an increase in intakes of vegetables and fruits in the UK. The WHO and Scottish Office have developed population dietary goals advocating a mean consumption of 400g a day or more. A variety of health promotion programmes in Europe and the United States have recommended consuming at least five portions of vegetables and fruits a day. It is estimated that achieving these levels of intake in the UK would represent a 60% increase on current consumption levels. For people in lower socioeconomic groups, a much larger increase would be required.

Until more is known about the precise effects of each antioxidant, and of other bioactive micronutrients present in foods of plant origin, it seems prudent to raise the intakes of antioxidant nutrients through increasing the consumption of vegetables and fruit rather than through widespread fortification of the diet or through vitamin supplements.

The challenge is to create and implement a sustained strategy and action plan to bridge the gap between the consistent recommendations on fruit and vegetables and the low intakes in the UK.

GLOSSARY

Dietary Reference Value (DRV) is a generic term for a range of figures which provide benchmarks for describing the adequacy of nutrient intake. COMA proposed three DRVs which reflect the biological variation in nutrient requirements in the population, as follows:

RNI   Reference Nutrient Intake. An amount which more than meets the needs of most people. Updated equivalent of the old Recommended Daily Amount.

EAR   Estimated Average Requirement. Average requirement of the population. By definition, it is more than enough for 50% of the population, and not enough for the other 50%.

LRNI   Lower Reference Nutrient Intake. The amount of the nutrient which is sufficient for the 3% of people in a population who have the lowest needs. Anyone regularly eating less than the LRNI may be at risk of deficiency.

References

1   Committee on Diet and Health, Food and Nutrition Board, National Research Council. 1989. *Diet and Health: Implications for Reducing Chronic Disease Risk*. Washington DC: National Academy Press.

2   United States Department of Health and Human Services. 1991. *Healthy People 2000: National Health Promotion and Disease Prevention Objectives. DHHS (PHS) Publication No. DHS-91-50213*. Washington DC: US Government Printing Office.

3   World Health Organization. 1990. *Diet, Nutrition and the Prevention of Chronic Diseases. WHO Technical Report Series 1990 (797)*. Geneva: World Health Organization.

4   The Scottish Office. 1993. *The Scottish Diet. Report of a Working Party to the Chief Medical Officer for Scotland*. Edinburgh: The Scottish Office Home and Health Department/HMSO Scotland.

5   Department of Health. 1994. *Nutritional Aspects of Cardiovascular Disease. Report of the Cardiovascular Review Group, Committee on Medical Aspects of Food Policy. Report on Health and Social Subjects 46*. London: HMSO.

6   Food and Nutrition Strategy Group. 1996. *Eating and Health – A Food and Nutrition Strategy for Northern Ireland*. Belfast: The Health Promotion Agency for Northern Ireland.

7   Ames BN, Shigenaga MK, Hagen TM. 1993. Oxidants, antioxidants and the degenerative diseases of aging. *Proceedings of the National Academy of Science USA;* 90: 7915-7922.

8   Ministry of Agriculture Fisheries and Food. 1988. *Food Portion Sizes. Second Edition*. London: HMSO.

9   Williams C. 1995. Healthy eating: clarifying advice about fruit and vegetables. *British Medical Journal;* 310: 1453-1455.

10 *The Food Pyramid Food Guide. Beyond the Basic 4*. United States Department of Agriculture, 1992.

11 Health Education Authority. 1994. *The Balance of Good Health*. London: Health Education Authority.

12 Professor P James. Personal communication.

13 Belizzi MC, Franklin MF, Duthie GG et al. 1994. Vitamin E and coronary heart disease: The European paradox. *European Journal of Clinical Nutrition;* 48: 822-831.

14 Gregory J, Foster K, Tyler H, Wiseman M for the Office of Population Censuses and Surveys. 1990. *The Dietary and Nutritional Survey of British Adults*. London: HMSO.

15 Williams C. 1997. In: *At Least Five a Day. Strategies to Increase Fruit and Vegetable Consumption*. London: National Heart Forum/The Stationery Office.

16 Billson H. 1993. *Eating Fruit and Vegetables. An Analysis of Fruit and Vegetable Consumption for the Dietary and Nutritional Survey of British Adults*. MSc Report. London: Centre for Human Nutrition, London School of Hygiene and Tropical Medicine.

17 Ministry of Agriculture, Fisheries and Food. 1995. *Household Food Consumption and Expenditure Survey. 1994. Annual Report of the National Food Survey Committee*. London: HMSO.

18 Ministry of Agriculture, Fisheries and Food. 1994. *The Dietary and Nutritional Survey of British Adults - Further Analysis*. London: HMSO.

19 Doyle W, Jenkins S, Crawford MA et al. 1994. Nutritional status of school children in an inner city area. *Archives of Diseases of Childhood;* 70 (5): 376-381.

20 Williams C, Ward P. 1993. *School Meals: Report of a Survey of Parents' Attitudes to the School Meals Service, and Weekday Dietary Habits of School Children in Seven Case Study Schools*. London: Consumers' Association.

21 Ministry of Agriculture, Fisheries and Food. 1991. *Household Food Consumption and Expenditure Survey. 1990. Annual Report of the National Food Survey Committee*. London: HMSO.

Professor Michael Marmot is an individual member of the National Heart Forum.

Acknowledgements

The authors of Chapters 5 and 6 thank Geoffrey Cannon and Alizon Draper of the World Cancer Research Fund (WCRF), for providing generous access to WCRF's extensive resource collection on diet and cancer.

Rich sources of beta-carotene, vitamin C and vitamin E

Beta-carotene

		portion size	
Vegetables	carrot	one, boiled (80g)	6mg
	spinach	boiled (90g)	3.5mg
	sweet potatoes	one, boiled (65g)	2.6mg
	spring greens	boiled (95g)	2.2mg
	pumpkin	65g	0.6mg
	watercress	quarter bunch (20g)	0.5mg
	tomato	one (85g)	0.5mg
	broccoli	85g	0.4mg
	lettuce	salad serving (30g)	0.1mg
Fruit	cantaloupe melon	slice (150g)	1.5mg
	apricot	one (40g)	0.2mg
	peach	one (110g)	0.1mg
Miscellaneous	butter	18g	0.1mg

Vitamin C

		portion size	
Fruit	blackcurrants, stewed	140g	161mg
	strawberries	10 (120g)	92mg
	orange	160g	86mg
	orange juice, long-life	glass (170ml)	77mg
	kiwi fruit	60g	35mg
	banana	100g	11mg
Vegetables	red pepper	160g	224mg
	Brussels sprouts	90g	54mg
	potatoes, new, boiled	175g	26mg
	broccoli, boiled	90g	20mg
	chips, home-made	180g/25g	16mg
	tomato, raw	one (85g)	14mg

Vitamin E

		portion size	
Oils	wheat germ oil	1 tablespoonful (11g)	5.4mg
	sunflower oil	1 tablespoonful (11g)	4.5mg
	rapeseed oil	1 tablespoonful (11g)	2.4mg
	soya, corn or groundnut oil	1 tablespoonful (11g)	1.8mg
Vegetables and fruits	blackberries	100g	2.4mg
	mango	160g	1.7mg
	spinach	average serving (90g)	1.5mg
	orange or grapefruit juice	glass (200ml)	1.4mg
Nuts and seeds	peanuts, plain	small pack (25g)	2.5 mg
	sunflower seeds	1 tablespoonful (14g)	3.8mg
	muesli	average serving (50g)	1.6mg
Miscellaneous	mayonnaise	1 tablespoonful (30g)	5.7mg
	salad cream	1 tablespoonful (30g)	3.1mg
	avocado	half (75g)	2.4mg
	sweet potatoes, boiled	average serving (120g)	5.3mg

Source: Holland B et al. 1992. *McCance and Widdowson's The Composition of Foods: Fifth Edition.* Cambridge: Royal Society of Chemistry and Ministry of Agriculture, Fisheries and Food.

Printed in the United Kingdom for The Stationery Office
Dd303143 3/97 C15 G559 10170